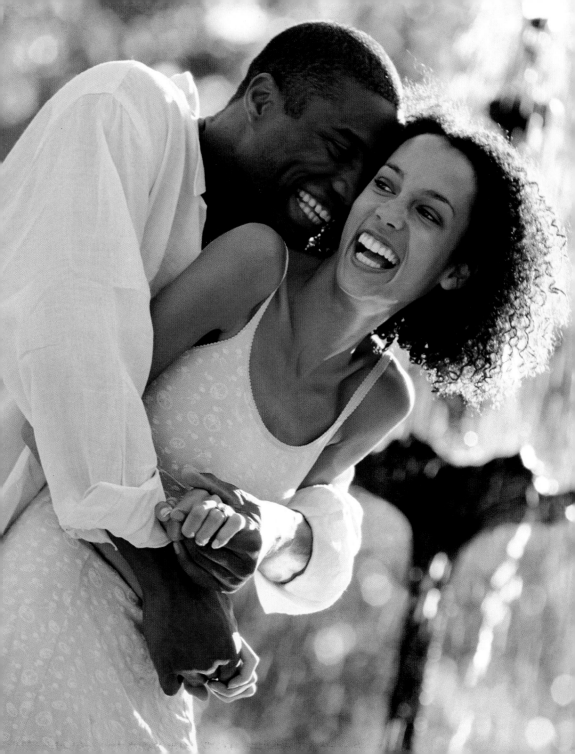

The Five-Minute Healer

EASY, NATURAL WAYS TO LOOK AND FEEL BETTER FAST

JANE ALEXANDER

A Fireside Book
Published by Simon & Schuster

New York   London   Sydney   Singapore

FIRESIDE
Rockefeller Center
1230 Avenue of the Americas
New York, NY 10020

Designed by Phil Gamble

Manufactured in Singapore

10 9 8 7 6 5 4 3 2 1

Note to readers
This publication contains the opinions and ideas of its author. It is intended
to provide helpful and informative material on the subjects addressed in the
publication. It is sold with the understanding that the author and publisher
are not engaged in rendering medical, health, psychological, or any other
kind of personal, professional services in the book. The reader should
consult his or her medical, health, or other competent professional before
adopting any of the suggestions in this book or drawing inferences from it.

The author and the publisher specifically disclaim all responsibility for any
liability, loss or risk, personal, or otherwise, which is incurred as a
consequence, directly or indirectly, of the use and application of any of the
contents of this book.

Library of Congress Cataloging-in-Publication Data is available.

ISBN 0-684-86945-4

ACKNOWLEDGMENTS
All photography/illustrations
by Gus Filgate, Dominic
Blackmore, Paul Forrester,
Iain Bagwell, Mark Preston
except: DigitalVision pp. 2,
8, 40, 41, 42, 43, 51, 112,
120, 142; ImageSource pp.
53, 80, 81, 82, 83;
PhotoDisc p 45; Tony Stone
Images pp. 54, 66, 104,
117, 128, 130, 134, 137,
144, 147.

Gaia Books would like to
thank Lynn Bresler, Gwen
Rigby, Dee Jones, Kate
Smith, Suzi Langhorne,
Dianne Rhule, Zoe Calvert,
Mark Bowden, Patrick
Jones, Kentaro Suyama,
Penny Markham, and
Louise Pickford.

How to use this book

Who doesn't want more energy? Who wouldn't love to feel bright and clear-headed, calm and focused throughout the day? The answer lies within this book. Simple techniques from natural therapies can keep us in optimum health and vitality. They can balance our energy, our life force, allowing us to calmly breeze through the stresses, strains, and demands of everyday life.

But what if you simply don't have the time to investigate which therapy would suit you best? What if you don't have the luxury of hours to spend in esoteric practices, extended exercise, or compli-cated diets? *The Five Minute Healer* has done all the work for you. It takes away all the research, all the decisions, all the dilemmas, leaving you with clear-cut, swift solutions – that really work.

Structured around the average working day, each chapter introduces natural and effective techniques to keep you well, energetic, and feeling great. Whether you have to negotiate rush-hour traffic or handle a difficult meeting, there are speedy solutions on hand. Whether you need to give yourself an instant boost

of energy or wind down after a day full of stresses, *The Five Minute Healer* has the answer. It gives the busy person everything needed to survive the modern world.

How you use this book is entirely up to you. You can dip into *The Five Minute Healer* as a quick-fix reference manual. When you feel your energy slumping or your stress levels rising, simply thumb through the book and find a suitable pick-me-up. However, if you want to go further, you can use the book as a complete lifestyle guide – a blueprint for healthy living. If you really want to get your life on track, your energy buzzing, and your body in tune with both mind and soul, take on board as many of the suggestions as you like. The more you try, the better you will feel!

Hopefully you will find the exercises and techniques in this book not only effective but fun as well. The key to making healthy habits is to find things that are enjoyable. Nobody wants to become a slave to their health – life is for enjoying! So I wish you good health, great energy, and a wonderful life.

Jane Alexander

Contents

How to use this book   5
Contents   6

PART ONE: GET UP AND GO!   8

CHAPTER ONE
A positive start   10

Fresh day, fresh start   12
Clear the cobwebs   13
Greet the day   14
Ground yourself   16
Jumpstart your body   18
Prepare for a difficult day   22
Be calm and centred   23
Dress for success   24

CHAPTER TWO
Power breakfasts and quick cures   26

Healthy eating   28
The energy breakfast   30
Smooth your way to health   32
Sickness and indigestion   34
Zap your hangover   36
Detox your body   37
Banish a cold   38

CHAPTER THREE
On the way to work   40

Your car as sanctuary   42
Save your spine   43
Let it out: sound stress busters   44
Stay alert   45
Banish road rage   46
Keep your cool   47
Waiting in line – keeping your cool   48
Balance your energy   50
Walk to success   51

PART TWO: WINNING AT WORK   52

CHAPTER FOUR
Your working space   54

Clearing clutter   56
Boost your career   58
Gain recognition   60
Combat sick office syndrome   62
Ease back and neck strain   64

CHAPTER FIVE
Easing physical and mental stress 66

Concentrate 68
Soothe eye strain 70
Instant refresher 72
You can do it 74
Combat shyness 76
Diffuse arguments 78
Power meetings 80
Creating rapport 82
Banish the blues 84
Overcome disappointment 86
Change your mood with music 88

CHAPTER SIX
Have a break 91

Refuel, revitalize 92
Recharge your batteries 94
Cool down 95
Rebalance body and mind 96
Let go of a bad morning 98
Gain total control 100

PART THREE: AFTER WORK 102

CHAPTER SEVEN
Leaving your work behind 104

Think ahead – plan for tomorrow 106
Cut the ties, make a break 108
Shift your mood 110
Banish a bad day 111

CHAPTER EIGHT
Time for yourself 112

Foods for moods 114
Prepare to party 116
Resolve your problems 118
Unleash your creativity 119
Discover your ideal exercise 120
Balance your diet 122
Conjure up romance 124
Go within and find peace 126

CHAPTER NINE
End of the day 128

Sleep soundly 130
Your pleasure zone 132
Create a safe space 134
Massage with a partner 136
Be soothed! 138
Sound sleep 140
Look younger 142
Banish bugs and flu 144
Arouse your sensuality 145
Enjoy super sex 146
Soothe insomnia 148
Sort out your psyche 150

Appendix: Recipes 152
Resources 154
Further reading 156
Index 158

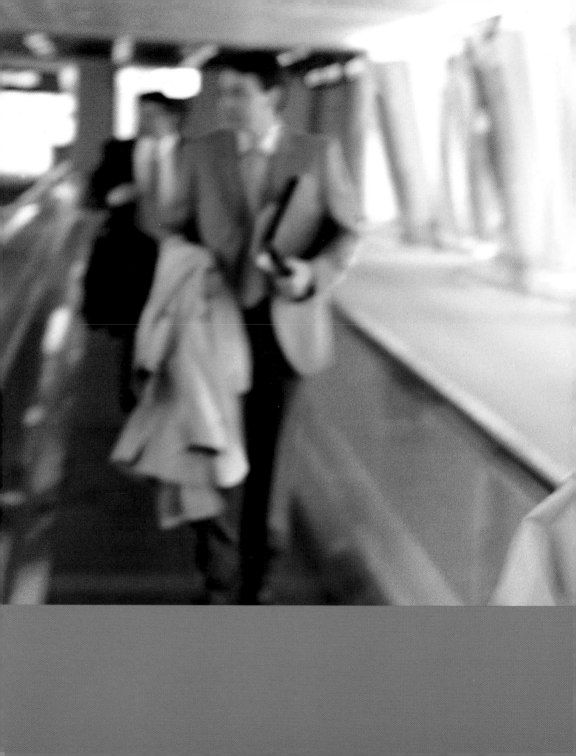

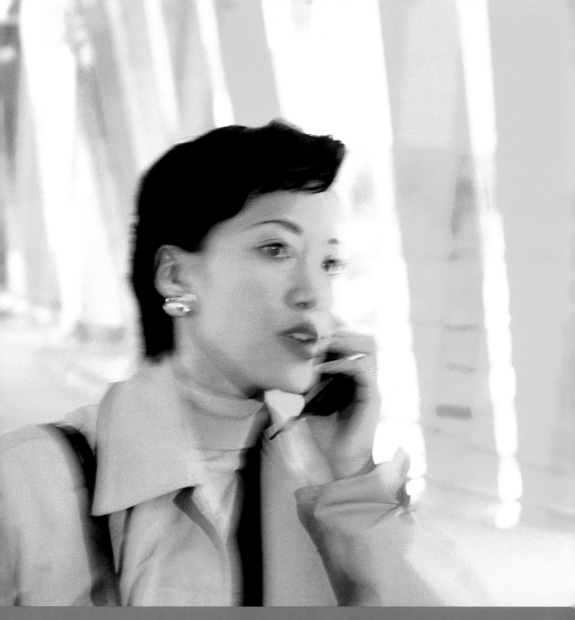

Part one: Get up and go!

Your first few minutes awake set the pattern for the whole day. Get it right and you'll sail through.

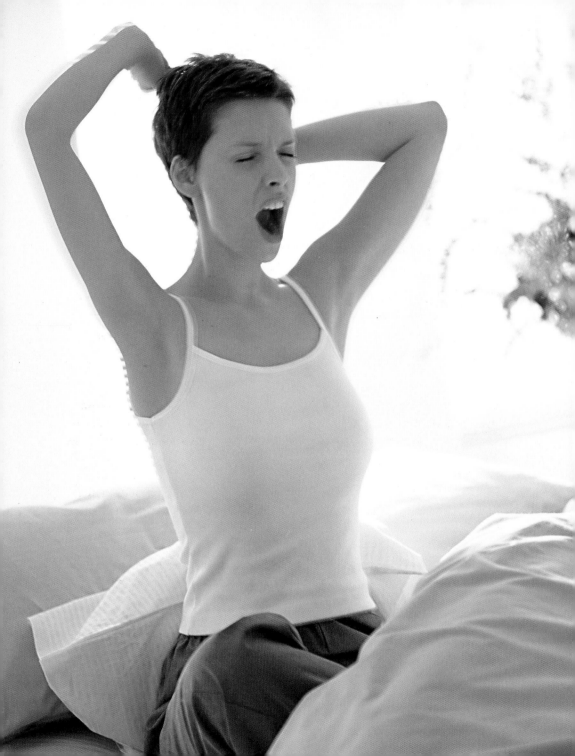

CHAPTER ONE

A positive start

Good morning! Another day, another fresh start – make the most of it. How you start each day is crucial. Your mood and attitude in the first few minutes of waking set the tone for the rest of the day. If you crawl out of bed, worrying about the day ahead, you are setting yourself up for misery. So start each day as you mean to go on – bright, enthusiastic, energized, and full of joy.

A good start to the day involves two essential factors. Firstly good movement. When you get out of bed after a long night of inactivity you need to get your body warmed and moving – to give your subtle energy, or chi, a lightning flash of vitality.

So we start with some stretching to shake off the cobwebs. Then you could wake yourself right up by greeting the sun with yoga or by bouncing on a rebounder while you watch the morning news. Send shivers of energy tingling down your spine with an invigorating bout of skin-brushing and power-showering. To complete your wake-up routine, chi kung exercises will ground you firmly, enabling you to face the day calmly and with confidence.

Secondly you have to consider your attitude. How do you want your day to go? Do you need to be calm and focused or full of power and authority? Are you faced with a difficult day of tough meetings or decisions? In this chapter, we look at ways to put your mind in gear for the day ahead.

Believe it or not but your choice of clothes can also help you achieve your goals for the day. Follow the colour advice to dress for success.

So greet the day with a smile and a stretch – however tough it might be. Remember that you and you alone have the power to make this day whatever you want of it. Seize the day!

Fresh day, fresh start

You've just woken up. Welcome to the start of a brand new day. What you do in the next five minutes can profoundly affect the whole day ahead. So start as you mean to go on.

MIND AND BODY WAKE-UP

1 *When you wake up don't leap out of bed – spend time becoming aware of your body. How does it feel?*
2 *Stretch your body, slowly flexing your arms up over your head and pushing your feet to the end of the bed.*
3 *Take your knees up to your chest and let them gently fall to one side of your body. Slowly turn your head and arms to face the opposite direction. You may find a few vertebrae crunch a little. Repeat on the other side.*
4 *Sit on the edge of the bed. Very gently, lower your right ear towards your right shoulder, then your left ear to your left shoulder. Repeat five times.*
5 *Now stand. Feel the strong, quiet power of the earth rising through your feet. Raise your arms and imagine the sun pouring in through the top of your head, filling you with confidence and optimism.*
6 *Bring your arms to waist level and gently swing them from side to side, allowing your body to twist gently from the waist. Visualize yourself becoming flexible enough to deal with everything the day will bring.*
7 *Bring your hands together, shut your eyes, and state your aim for the day. It could be something like, "I will bring vision, truth, and kindness to my working day." Choose your own but make it meaningful.*

NOTES
★ *Don't stretch if you wake up cold – you will need to warm your muscles first.*
★ *Check with your physician before doing this exercise if you have any neck or back problems.*

Clear the cobwebs

Give yourself a wake-up call by turning your morning
shower into a mini power-spa. Skin brushing is one
of the simplest yet most effective techniques for
recharging your body and improving your health.
It stimulates the lymphatic system (an essential part
of the body's immune system) and helps you expel
toxins. Some claim that it also breaks down cellulite,
and it will definitely bring a clean, healthy glow to
your skin. Follow it with a bracing shower and some
positive affirmations and you'll be set for the day.

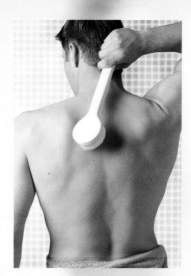

SKIN BRUSHING

1 *Use a long-handled natural bristle brush.*
2 *Brushing should be done on dry skin, before
showering. Follow these steps to brush over your whole
body for at least five minutes, until your skin glows.*
3 *Start by brushing your feet, toes, and soles. Then
brush up the front and back of your legs, with smooth,
long strokes. You should always brush towards the
groin area (a site of major lymph nodes).*
4 *Next brush your buttocks and lower back,
brushing towards the armpits (where there are
more major lymph nodes).*
5 *Now brush up both sides of your arms, from
hands (including the palms) to armpits.*
6 *Continue brushing across your shoulders and
down your chest towards the heart. Women
should not brush their nipples. Then brush the
back of your neck, with downward strokes.*
7 *Use a circular movement to brush your
abdominal area, avoiding the genitals. Brush in a
clockwise direction to stimulate the colon.*

Greet the day

The Sun Salute or Salutation to the Sun is the perfect way to kickstart your day. It's a well-known yoga routine which massages the internal organs as well as stretching every muscle in the body, thus increasing flexibility.

HOW TO PERFORM THE SUN SALUTE
Start by doing the whole set once and gradually build up to twelve sets. With practice you will be able to move smoothly from one position to the next. You may find it helpful to tape the instructions.

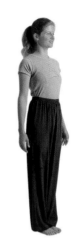

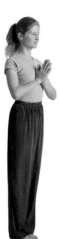

10 *Return to the standing position, big toes touching, arms by your sides. Exhale as you look straight ahead and bring your hands together.*

1 *Stand with your feet together, big toes touching, arms by your sides. Tuck your chin in, look straight ahead, and keep your shoulders relaxed.*

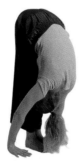

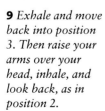

9 *Exhale and move back into position 3. Then raise your arms over your head, inhale, and look back, as in position 2.*

8 *Inhale and return to position 4, this time with your left leg stretched backwards.*

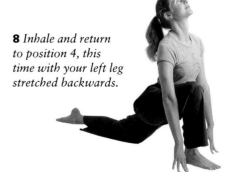

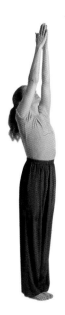

2 *Bring your arms up over your head, inhaling slowly and deeply. As you finish inhaling, put your palms together and look back at your thumbs.*

3 *Exhale as you bend forwards, placing your hands on the floor beside your feet. Touch your head to your knees (you may have to bend your knees slightly at first).*

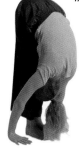

4 *Inhale deeply and stretch your right leg back to an extended lunge. Tilt your head backwards to stretch your back.*

5 *Exhale and push your left leg back to join your right leg. Rise on to your toes. Support yourself on your hands, keeping your arms straight and shoulder-width apart. Your head, back, and legs should be in a straight line. Breathe slowly and deeply.*

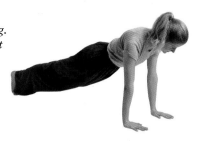

7 *Inhale and push until your arms are straight, with hands on the floor in front of you. Bend backwards and look upwards. Then exhale and return to position 5 again via position 6.*

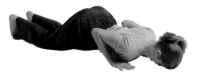

6 *Exhale again and lower yourself to the floor. Keep your abdomen raised. Only your toes, knees, hands, chest, and forehead should touch the floor.*

Ground yourself

When you need to keep your feet firmly on the ground, to keep a steady head and solid nerves, turn to chi kung. These apparently simple exercises have profound effects: improved concentration and creativity, increased vitality, and improved ability to cope with stress.

CAUTION
Chi kung is very powerful. If you have a chest problem perform these exercises carefully. If you have a blood pressure problem or a heart condition don't hold your breath. Always consult your doctor if you are in doubt.

THE STARTING POSITION
This basic posture for chi kung is also used as a starting pose for other exercises in this book. It brings all the organs into alignment and helps you become aware of your entire body.
1 *Stand with your feet shoulder-width apart. Find your natural balance, with weight neither too far forwards nor too far back.*
2 *Feel how your feet are relaxed where they touch the floor – heel, toes, and along the outer edge.*
3 *Relax your knees over your feet.*
4 *Relax your lower back, stomach, and buttocks.*
5 *Relax and round your shoulders slightly, allowing your chest to hollow.*

6 *Imagine that the top of your head is tied by your hair to the roof. Feel your head floating freely. Then relax your tongue, mouth, and jaw.*
7 *Remain in this position, hands hanging loosely by your sides, for a few minutes.*
8 *Focus your mind on the five elements. For Earth, imagine the feeling of weight and rootedness; for Water, looseness and fluidity; for Air, lightness and transparency; for Fire, sparkle; and for Space, envisage the space within each joint, muscle, breath, and in your mind.*
9 *During these chi kung exercises, keep your mind restful by gently bringing it back to your posture.*

DRAGON STAMPING

*This exercise helps to calm
the mind and, if performed
every morning, helps you
become focused and
energized for the day ahead.
Make sure you are breathing
out as you rise and in as you
return – it's very easy to get
it the wrong way round,
which is far less effective.*
1 *Stand in the starting
position (page 16).*

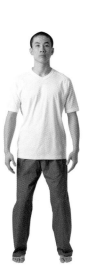
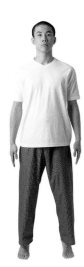

2 *Exhale and rise slowly
onto your tiptoes. Stretch
your body upwards, keeping
your abdomen relaxed. At
the same time stretch your
arms downwards, with
fingers pointed.*
3 *Lower your heels slowly as
you inhale and relax. Repeat
the sequence at least five
times.*

SUPPORTING THE SKY

*This connects you with the sky
and earth – combining
inspiration and
grounded-
ness.*
1 *Stand in the
starting position
(page 16).*
2 *Breathe in and
sweep your
hands up past
your abdomen
then your chest,
palms facing
your body. As
they pass your
face, roll them
so the palms face
up to the sky.*

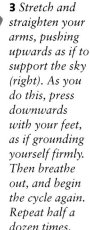

3 *Stretch and
straighten your
arms, pushing
upwards as if to
support the sky
(right). As you
do this, press
downwards
with your feet,
as if grounding
yourself firmly.
Then breathe
out, and begin
the cycle again.
Repeat half a
dozen times.*

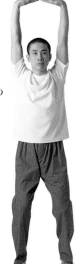

4 *This time,
instead of
pressing down,
rise slowly to
stand on tiptoe
(right) and fully
stretch your arms
and legs.*

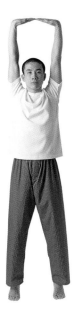

Jumpstart your body

If you're really pushed for time in the morning, take your exercise while you're watching or listening to the breakfast news! Bouncing on a rebounder (a small trampoline) is a simple and effective way to jumpstart your body, increasing energy and vitality and giving you a stress-free start to the day.

CAUTION
★ *Check with a medical practitioner if you suffer from: heart disease, dizziness, chest pains, osteoporosis, arthritis or joint pain, prolapsed uterus, detached retina, or phlebitis.*

WARM-UP
Stand in the middle of the rebounder with your feet shoulder-width apart, in the chi kung starting position (see page 16). Your breathing should be deep and relaxed.

Start bouncing gently, without lifting your feet from the rebounder. Keep your knees relaxed. Then move into a gentle walking pace. Once your feet are moving smoothly and rhythmically, let your arms swing gently. Your left arm should swing forwards as your right heel rises and vice versa.

AEROBIC WORKOUT

Now you have warmed up, it's time to move into some high-intensity exercise, working your muscles and increasing your pulse rate.

Spotty dog

Jump as you slide one foot forwards and one back alternately. Swing your arm opposite to your leg – your left foot and right arm go forwards together. The movement looks a bit like cross-country skiing.

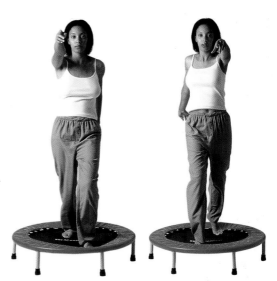

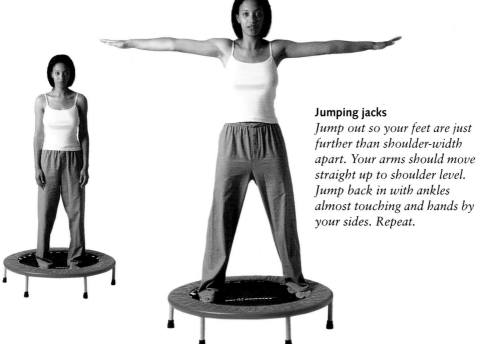

Jumping jacks

Jump out so your feet are just further than shoulder-width apart. Your arms should move straight up to shoulder level. Jump back in with ankles almost touching and hands by your sides. Repeat.

19

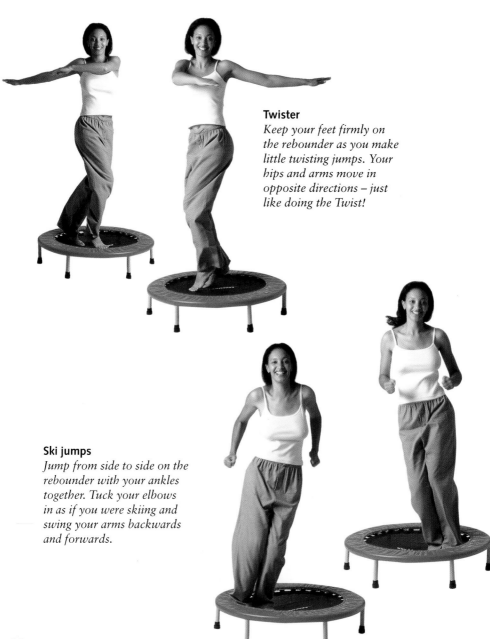

Twister
Keep your feet firmly on the rebounder as you make little twisting jumps. Your hips and arms move in opposite directions – just like doing the Twist!

Ski jumps
Jump from side to side on the rebounder with your ankles together. Tuck your elbows in as if you were skiing and swing your arms backwards and forwards.

Jogging
Lean slightly forwards and move from a walk into a jog. Once you have found your rhythm, kick your heels up behind you and swing your arms.

CAUTION
★ *Do not bounce on a full stomach, when suffering from colds or viruses, or when you are overly tired.*
★ *Do not bounce in slippery shoes or socks. Either wear well-fitting trainers or bounce in bare feet.*

Knee lifts
Lift your knees in front of you, alternately, pointing your toes. Pull your arms from above your head down over your raised knee.

Cool down and stretch
Bring your heartbeat down gently by walking for a few minutes, as in the warm-up. Make sure you drink plenty of fresh water. Rebounding is hard exercise.

Prepare for a difficult day

There are some days we all dread. This "swish" technique, which comes from NLP (neuro-linguistic programming), can help you turn past failures into present-day success.

SWISH TECHNIQUE

1 *Identify what behaviour you would like to change. Close your eyes and decide on a cue picture – think about what you see just before you start your habitual behaviour. How do you feel in this state? Feel it as unpleasantly as possible. Maybe it's you feeling, and looking, small and insignificant.*
2 *Create a picture of how you would like to look and feel instead – in your ideal confident, energized state. Make it powerful. You'll feel a frisson of energy when you hit the right picture.*
3 *Imagine your unpleasant cue picture on a large movie screen – big, colourful, and clear – it's a horrible picture.*
4 *Place the picture of the new confident you on the screen in the bottom left-hand corner. This picture is small and black and white.*
5 *Now you can begin to "swish." Swiftly bring up the small positive picture until it fills the whole screen, completely obliterating the negative picture. As it expands, it becomes bright, multicoloured, and clear. The negative picture shrinks away into a corner, becoming small and dark.*
6 *Open your eyes, stamp your feet and shake your limbs. Clear your mind of the picture.*
7 *Now repeat steps 4 and 5 five times – as quickly as possible, stopping and blanking the screen between each swish.*

PROGRAMMING FOR SUCCESS
The negative picture should become harder and harder to keep in your mind. By building up the positive pattern, you are programming yourself for success. Reinforce your confidence by swishing just before you go into the difficult situation and notice the difference!

Be calm and centred

Try to make time for five minutes of quiet meditation before you leave for work. It stills the mind, combats stress, and mentally prepares you for the day ahead.

MEDITATION EXERCISE

1 *Sit in any position that feels comfortable and close your eyes. Keep your head upright, shoulders relaxed.*
2 *Start to breathe steadily and deeply. Don't try to influence your breathing too much – just notice it for a few minutes.*
3 *Now start your mantra by intoning a deep "OH" sound that comes from the back of your mouth and throat. Bring the sound forwards in your mouth, opening your mouth wider, as the sound seamlessly shifts into a slightly higher-pitched "AH." Finally close your lips and hum the sound "MMM." Feel it vibrate on your lips.*
4 *Repeat twice more. Take it very slowly – make the sounds as rich and vibrant as you can, and extend them for as long as you can.*
5 *How do you feel now? Do you feel different in any way? Can you feel any tingling of subtle energy, or chi, in your body or head?*

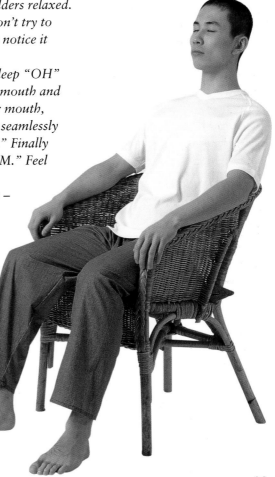

Meditate with your head upright, shoulders relaxed, and with a deep and steady breath.

Dress for success

Does it really matter what colour suit you wear for work? Could your choice of jacket mean the difference between success and second best? According to colour therapists, the colours of our workwear can affect everything from our mood and confidence to how people perceive us. Match the colours you wear to the task in hand and your day should turn out just right.

THE POWER SUIT

When you need to command respect and attention choose the classic black suit. Black gives you confidence and conveys power. However, combine it with other colours for maximum impact – otherwise it can make you seem aloof, unapproachable, and intimidating. Of course, that might be the desired effect but if you really want to head for the top, combine your black suit with red accessories (see right).

Standard alternatives to the black suit are not so successful. Grey signifies you are cool, calm, and in control but that you are not a major league player.

Brown can make you appear rather fixed and static. It is useful if you feel nervous and need security but avoid it if you need to turn on the power.

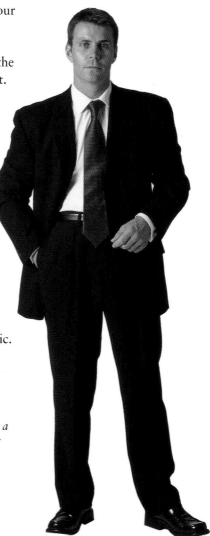

Look like you mean business in a black suit accented with a tie or shirt in a colour sympathetic to your personality. See chart opposite for some ideas.

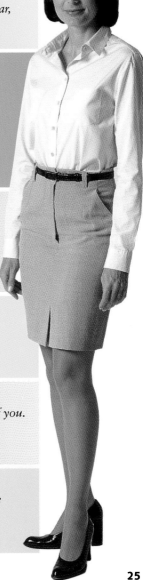

BE CREATIVE WITH ORANGE

If you work with creative ideas surround yourself with orange hues. Orange is a colour of warmth, vitality, and creativity – it stimulates the brain to try new ideas, new ways of working. Apricot, in particular, increases creative ideas and artistic awareness.

GRAB ATTENTION WITH RED

Red pushes you to the front – it is energetic, vibrant, and screams confidence. Go for red if you need to make an impact.

Red makes you feel adventurous. If you are dreading a meeting or task, if you feel lacking in energy or in low spirits, give yourself a push with red. It doesn't have to be a full red-on-red ensemble, even a scarf or tie would help your confidence.

BE CALM WITH BLUE

Blue is ideal when you need to introduce calm and centredness into your working day. It is also useful if you are expecting arguments at work – blue soothes the situation.

BE CONFIDENT WITH YELLOW

Yellow boosts self-esteem. It is a friendly, communicative colour. Use it (in small amounts) when you want to stimulate conversation and encourage dialogue.

BE FASCINATING WITH TURQUOISE

Turquoise draws people towards you, and makes them think well of you. It is a useful colour to wear if you're giving a presentation or a talk.

BE LOVING IN PINK

Pink is loving, warm, and caring, making it a useful choice for those in the caring professions. Wear some pink for occasions when you need to pacify, or to show you are not a threat.

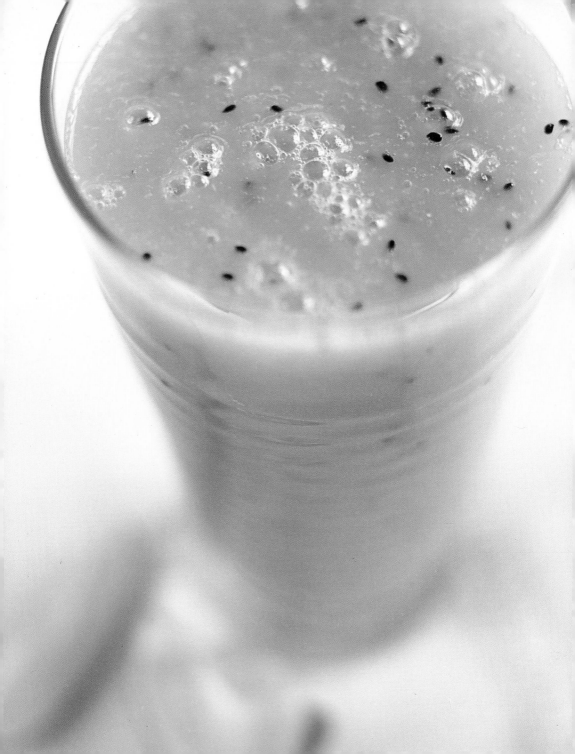

CHAPTER TWO

Power breakfasts and quick cures

There's never enough time in the morning. So simple things like breakfast tend to be forgotten or eaten on the run. Yet spare yourself just five minutes to eat something tasty and energizing, and it will set you up for the day.

Once you've kickstarted your body into action with some kind of exercise, the next step is to stoke up with your first fuel of the day. A good breakfast is essential for supplying you with the long-lasting energy you'll need throughout the day. If you choose your start-up meal with care and eat it without hurrying, you will power through the morning without a worry.

If you are one of those people who can't face eating a large breakfast, don't panic. This chapter will give you plenty of options for foods for healthy eating and drinks packed with nutrients – and they are delicious too!

We will also take a look at how to zap common health problems. You've woken up with a cold? You'll discover how to treat your symptoms with supplements, homeopathic remedies, or good old-fashioned steam, to banish the cold and help yourself feel human.

You're feeling sick with an upset stomach after overindulging in rich foods the night before? Herbs and homeopathy can help reduce your nausea or indigestion, so you can survive the day. And if you're facing a day's work with a hangover from the previous night (and, let's face it, who hasn't?), there are some life-savers to make the world seem a more bearable place.

So there's absolutely no excuse for not getting off to a great start.

LEFT: Kiwi and lime smoothie. For more smoothie recipes see pages 152–153

Healthy eating

It's tough to eat well when you're busy. But eating healthily need not be a chore: the essence of healthy eating is simplicity itself. Find out what food suits you and plan for it – food is not a convenience but a vital part of your life.

Just follow these good-guy and bad-guy rules and improve your diet – and your health – almost overnight. And remember, there are cooking techniques, such as steaming, poaching, grilling, and stir-frying, to suit your hectic lifestyle. They don't take much time yet provide you with nourishing meals.

THE GOOD GUYS – FOR HEALTHY EATING

■ The food you eat should be organic, fresh, seasonal, and grown as locally as possible. Food that is not organic is often sprayed to combat pests and diseases, or treated artificially to improve its look and to give it a longer shelf life. If you cannot avoid eating nonorganic fruit and vegetables, make sure you peel the skin first.

■ Make sure you include the following three elements in your diet. First, as much fresh fruit and vegetables as possible – at least five portions every day. Second, plenty of complex carbohydrates – brown rice, millet, oats, potatoes, wholemeal pasta and bread. And third, some good protein, such as pulses, nuts, lean white meat, fish, and soy bean products.

■ Drink at least 3 pints (2 litres) of fresh mineral water each day.

■ Add plenty of fresh herbs and spices to your food – they have potent health benefits.

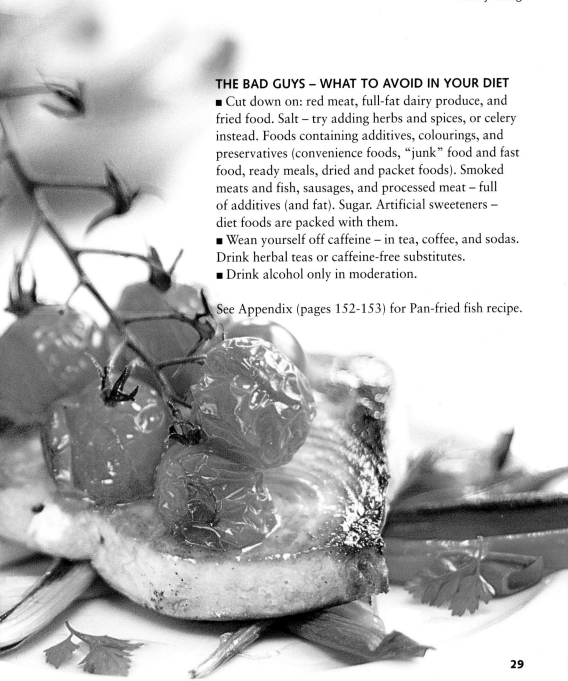

THE BAD GUYS – WHAT TO AVOID IN YOUR DIET

■ Cut down on: red meat, full-fat dairy produce, and fried food. Salt – try adding herbs and spices, or celery instead. Foods containing additives, colourings, and preservatives (convenience foods, "junk" food and fast food, ready meals, dried and packet foods). Smoked meats and fish, sausages, and processed meat – full of additives (and fat). Sugar. Artificial sweeteners – diet foods are packed with them.

■ Wean yourself off caffeine – in tea, coffee, and sodas. Drink herbal teas or caffeine-free substitutes.

■ Drink alcohol only in moderation.

See Appendix (pages 152-153) for Pan-fried fish recipe.

The energy breakfast

Do you skip breakfast because you're simply too busy? Or you're trying to lose weight? Don't! Eat a good breakfast and you will be giving your body and mind the fuel to power it right through the morning – and well into the afternoon.

EAT FOR ENERGY

Try one of these breakfast menus to give you a good balance of protein, fat, and carbohydrate:

Oatmeal porridge with milk or soya milk (provides slow-releasing carbohydrate). Stir in chopped almonds (protein and "good" fat), and sultanas (for sweetness – to avoid sugar).

Oatmeal soaked overnight in soy milk. In the morning, mix with more soy milk to taste and add sunflower seeds and dried fruit.

Avocado smoothie with soy milk and fresh fruit (blend together one large avocado, 2 teaspoons soy milk, and one cup of ice).

Wholemeal toast with peanut butter (low in sugar and salt), or use almond or sunflower-seed butter.

Baked beans (no added sugar and salt) on wholemeal toast with polyunsaturated fat spread. Add a piece of fresh fruit or fruit salad in summer, or a dish of stewed fruit sprinkled with cinnamon in winter.

A glass of fruit juice. Add a cup of coffee substitute with soy milk (e.g. Barleycup, dandelion coffee, Caro).

A cup of herbal tea (fennel and peppermint settle the digestion), or cinnamon tea to warm you in winter.

See Appendix (pages 152–153) for the recipes of Oatmeal porridge (main), Baked beans (inset bottom), and Avocado smoothie (inset top).

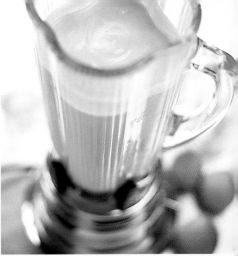

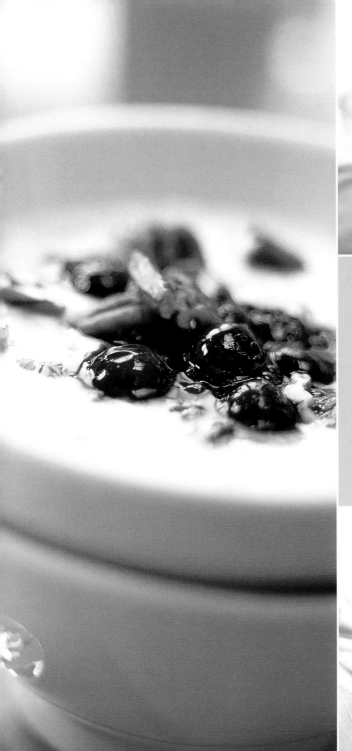

AVOID

★ *Carbohydrate-only breakfasts, such as breakfast cereals, which all contain sugar. This raises your blood sugar level quickly and then lets it plummet, leaving you feeling hungry and tired.*

★ *The classic "fry-up" – too much fat will make you sluggish and is terrible for your heart.*

★ *Sugar and coffee – stimulants that set your pulse racing, making you feel stressed. Coffee also takes the antistress mineral magnesium from your body.*

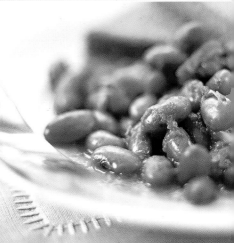

Smooth your way to health

Smoothies are the ultimate health breakfast packed in a glass. Brimming with vitamins, minerals, and phytonutrients (healing micronutrients derived from plants), these are drinks that really pack a health punch.

Health experts advise us to take at least five servings daily of fruit and vegetables because this will cut our risk of cancer by half. The drinks on these pages will give you your full daily requirement in one drink.

For the best effect, always make each serving fresh and serve it straight from the blender. Fruits and vegetables lose their nutrient power within a few hours of being peeled and crushed.

TIPS
- Quick and easy to prepare.
- Put your blender on the highest setting and whip the ingredients, together with a handful of ice cubes, until smooth and creamy.
- Use fruits and vegetables that are fresh, organic, seasonal, and locally grown – if you possibly can.
- Substitute the cold smoothies with warm, spicy milk in winter, or if you suffer from a sluggish metabolism or poor circulation.

See Appendix (pages 152–153) for the recipes for Summer Berry Attack (near right), Carrot Surprise (centre), and Tropical Delight (far right).

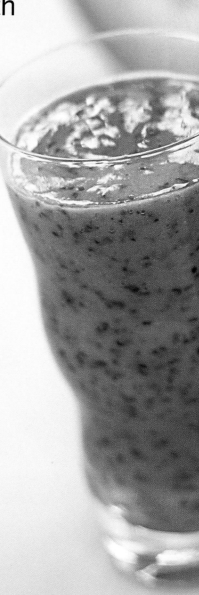

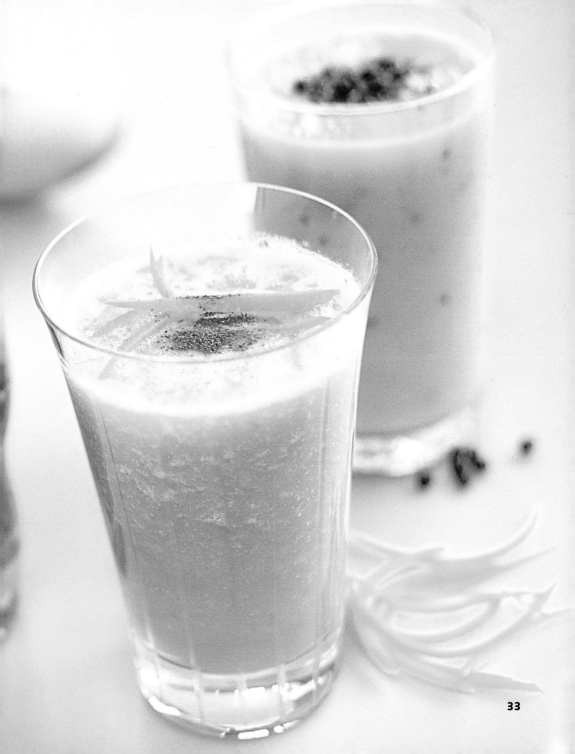

Sickness and indigestion

Last night was great – you had the most wonderful meal, washed down with a fair amount of alcohol. But this morning you feel terrible – nausea, heartburn, and wind threaten to make the day a misery. Try the following to ease the discomfort.

HOMEOPATHY

Homeopathy remedies are available from pharmacies and healthfood stores in different potencies, labelled 6c, 30c, etc. Choose the remedy from this list that matches your symptoms. Take one 30c tablet every hour for four doses.

■ **Nux vomica:** for sour taste, nausea, difficult belching of gas, weight and pain in the stomach.

■ **Arsenicum album:** for great thirst, nausea, retching, or after overeating or drinking, heartburn, burning pains, worse between midnight and 2a.m.

■ **Ipecacuanha:** for nausea after indigestible food, moist mouth, excess saliva, face pale and twitching, hiccups, a feeling as if stomach hanging down.

HERBALISM

Herbalism uses herbs to treat illness and restore the body to a state of balance.

■ Drink herbal teas: catnip, ginger, fennel, chamomile, peppermint. Add a few crushed fenugreek seeds and fresh parsley, too.

■ Take a quarter of a cup of aloe vera juice on an empty stomach.

■ Charcoal tablets help to absorb gas. Take them in between meals and separately from any supplements. Do not, however, use them on a regular basis since they interfere with the absorption of nutrients.

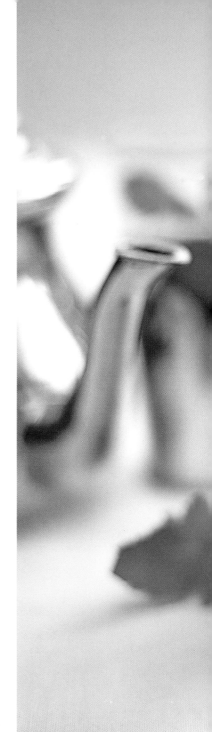

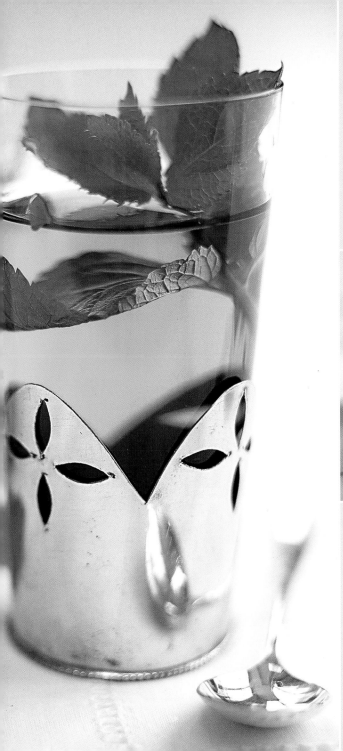

CAUTION
★ *Peppermint can reduce milk flow, so use with caution if breastfeeding.*
★ *Avoid ginger if you suffer from gastric ulcers.*
★ *Avoid fenugreek if you are diabetic, fennel if you're epileptic.*
★ *Seek advice from a herbalist before using these herbs.*

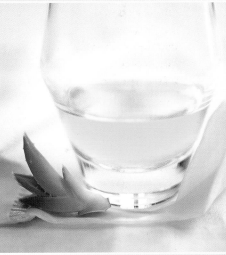

OTHER ADVICE
★ *If stress or anxiety is at the bottom of your problem, consider incorporating meditation (see page 23) into your daily routine. The balancing powers of yoga would also help (see pages 14–15).*
★ *Incorporate exercise into your daily routine.*

Zap your hangover

In a perfect world, of course, we wouldn't have hangovers. But life isn't perfect, is it? The easiest way to avoid hangovers is to be sensible the night before. But if you didn't have the presence of mind to do so, try these morning-after helpers.

■ A large glass of fresh, unsweetened, orange or grapefruit juice plus a good-quality multivitamin and mineral supplement – take the dose recommended on the packet.
■ A hot bath with two drops each of lavender and juniper, one drop of rosemary essential oil in the water.
■ Mix one drop each of fennel and juniper essential oils into one pint of warm water. Soak cotton pads in the solution, and place them on your forehead, temples, and liver area.
■ A cup of peppermint tea to soothe the stomach.
■ A simple wholesome breakfast: honey, on yogurt with a sprinkling of wheatgerm, or on porridge, followed by dry rye toast.

> **HOMEOPATHY**
> *Homeopathy has some excellent hangover cures. Remedies from pharmacies or healthfood stores will be labelled with the potency. Take the 6c potency of the remedy from this list that most closely matches your symptoms.*
> ★ *Nux vomica: head aches and the victim feels "dull, dizzy and irritable."*
> ★ *Pulsatilla: if hangover is due to rich food as well as alcohol.*
> ★ *Sulphur: excessive flatulence and nervous exhaustion, particularly following solitary drinking.*
> ★ *Kali bichrom: for beer drinkers who suffer nausea and vomiting.*

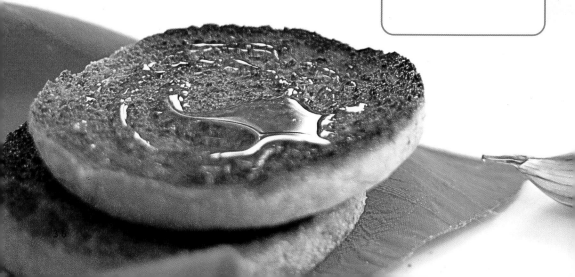

36

Detox your body

Stodgy meals and foods can clog the lymphatic system. When this system becomes blocked, toxins cannot be released effectively from the body. The build-up puts strain on the liver, kidneys, digestive, and immune systems.

The Liver Flush drink can help take the load off your lymph, helping to flush out toxins from the liver, cleansing the gall-bladder, kidneys, and intestinal tract.

IMPORTANT

If you have gall stones or a history of gall stones, seek specialist advice before taking this drink. Do not take it if you are pregnant or breastfeeding.

LIVER FLUSH

3–4 tablespoons of pure cold-pressed olive or almond oil, 6–8 tablespoons of freshly squeezed lemon juice, 3–6 cloves of garlic, and freshly grated ginger to taste. Blend all the ingredients in a blender until frothy. Drink immediately. Don't let the ingredients put you off – you soon get used to it!

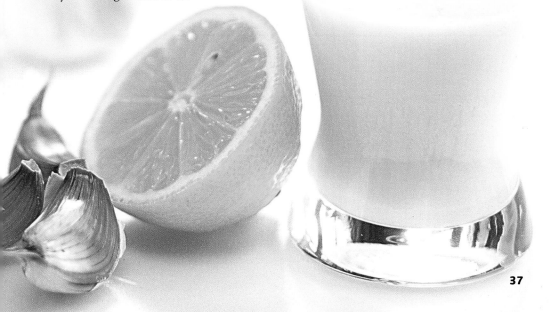

Banish a cold

You've woken up with a sore throat, thick head, and a stuffy nose. Yes, it's a cold. But you've got a meeting in an hour… . Try a remedy from these two pages – they could zap your cold altogether or, at the very least, make you feel more comfortable throughout the day.

SUPPLEMENTS
At the first sign of a cold, take the following together:
■ Buffered (nonacidic) vitamin C: take 5,000–15,000 mg daily for the duration of the cold only. Divide the dose through the day. This dose sounds very high but don't be alarmed – you will know if you are taking too much because your bowels will become loose. If this happens, lower the dose
■ A good-quality multivitamin and mineral plus an antioxidant complex – a blend of vitamins and minerals to boost immune function.
■ Echinacea – a herb that boosts immune function: 10 drops of the tincture two or three times a day.
■ A zinc lozenge (from food stores) every three hours – or follow instructions on the packet. Do not take more than 100 mg of zinc daily (include the zinc in other supplements you may be taking).

CAUTION
★ *Large doses of vitamin C, such as those recommended here, affect estrogen levels. Use additional forms of birth control if you take the contraceptive pill.*

STEAM
Put five drops of eucalyptus essential oil in a bowl of hot water. Place a towel over your head and the bowl. Slowly and carefully breathe in the steam.

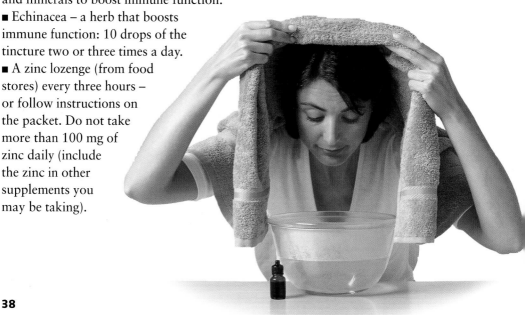

HOMEOPATHY

The right homeopathic remedy is the best chance of halting your cold in its tracks. But make sure the symptoms match exactly. Use these remedies in the 6c potency, available from pharmacies and healthfood stores.

REMEDY	SYMPTOMS
ACONITE	*The first remedy to think of the moment you feel a cold coming on. Cold comes on suddenly, often after exposure to cold winds. High fever; restless and anxious; runny nose. Feels better in fresh air.*
BRYONIA	*Cold starts in the nose but swiftly moves to the throat and chest with a dry, painful cough. Irritable; want to be left alone. Very thirsty for long drinks.*
NATRUM MURIATICUM (NAT MUR)	*Cold starts with sneezing. Copious clear or white discharge and maybe cold sores. Worse in fresh air and on exertion. Prefer to be left alone. Lose sense of taste completely.*
BELLADONNA	*Sudden onset but face (particularly cheeks) is bright red with dilated pupils. Every movement hurts; bad headache; blocked nose. Crave darkness, quiet, and warmth. Throat is red and sore. Crave lemon juice.*
GELSEMIUM	*Use early on in a cold. If you catch it early, gelsemium can break up a cold quicker than any other remedy. Symptoms start more slowly. Classic "hot and cold" with hot fever and cold chills up and down the spine. Head feels full. Great tiredness and weakness. Lack of thirst. Shivery and unable to get warm. Useful for summer colds and those brought on in unseasonably warm weather.*
ALLIUM CEPA	*Use when you have a runny nose with lots of mucus. Also your eyes, lips, and nostrils are red and sore with a slight burning sensation.*

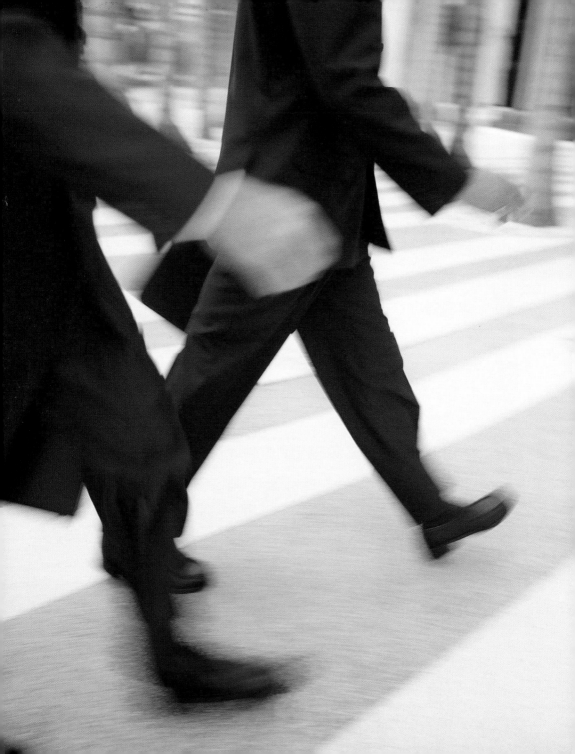

CHAPTER THREE

On the way to work

Few of us are lucky enough to work within a five-minute stroll of the office. Whether you travel to work in a car or by public transport, your inbound journey is always going to have the potential of being a source of stress and tension. Traffic jams, crazy drivers, overcrowded trains, and buses that arrive late if at all – it's enough to make you scream.

But keep your cool. In this chapter we look at ways to make your journey, if not pleasant, at least palatable. You'll learn how to turn your car into a peaceful, personal sanctuary.

When the traffic jams get worse and tension mounts, breathing exercises, as well as singing and chanting, will help you release stress and keep you calm behind the wheel. Techniques for staying focused as you drive, along with hints on posture to keep you sitting comfortably, take some of the strain out of long-distance driving.

If you travel regularly by public transport, each journey can become a mini-meditation when you learn how

to use simple techniques such as deep breathing and chi kung postures. Aura shielding visualization will help you to keep the crowds out of your own personal space, while discreet jin shin jyutsu exercises will balance and revitalize your energies.

You can make use of every step of your journey – from waiting in line to walking up the escalator. There is even a technique to reduce jet lag for you if you happen to commute by plane!

Enjoy your journey to work and remember that every journey (however small) is symbolic of our larger journey through life. Try to make yours meaningful.

Your car as sanctuary

The first step to stress-free commuting is to transform your car into a personal sanctuary – a pleasant comforting ease-zone. A five-minute clean and clear out is all it takes.

★ *Protect yourself: hang a small silver ball from your reversing mirror with a piece of red ribbon. According to feng shui, this will help deflect harmful energy. Maybe fix a favourite spiritual symbol on your dashboard. In some countries it's common to have a figure of the Virgin Mary. But you could choose a Buddha, a Star of David, a goddess, or your power animal.*

★ *Choose your music carefully to put you in the right frame of mind for driving – neither too aggressive nor too soporific. Talking books give you the opportunity to "read" a classic or laugh with a favourite comedian. Or start the day with words of wisdom from a self-help tape. Steer clear, however, of any tapes that contain deep relaxation exercises or self-hypnosis. Keep all your tapes and CDs in a tidy container.*

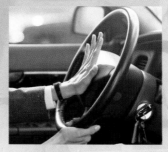

★ *Clear the clutter: clear out all the old newspapers, empty take-out cartons, coffee mugs, children's toys.*
★ *Clean thoroughly: put a few drops of grapefruit essential oil into your hoover bag and vacuum. Add a few drops of lemon and rosemary oils to a bowl of water and wash the mats. Polish the dashboard, using any of the above oils on your duster.*

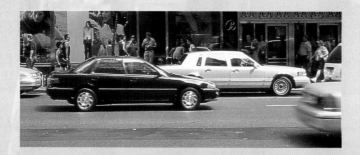

★ *Pack a spiritual emergency kit. A special book; feel-good essential oils and tissues to put them on; photos of loved ones; healthy snacks; mineral water; a cartoon to make you smile.*

Save your spine

Car seats are designed for safety, not your postural health. The Alexander Technique trains you in good posture – try these tips to save your spine every time you get into your car.

★ *Adjust your position so you don't have to stretch for the pedals – but don't hang over the wheel either. Your hands should be held at the "ten-to-two" position, resting lightly but firmly on the wheel.*

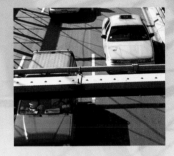

★ *Keep your seat upright and sit well back in your seat, making contact with the whole of your back. Try putting a wedge in the small of your back to prevent you from sinking right back.*

★ *Before you get into your car, take a moment to stand still. Let your body lengthen as if you were being gently held by a string from the top of your head. Feel your shoulders relax downwards, away from your ears. Feel your feet standing solidly on the ground. Let your mind become calm and centred.*
★ *Get into the car slowly and consciously. Sit down with both feet outside the car. Then mindfully swing both feet into the car.*

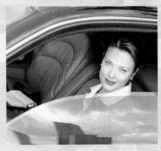

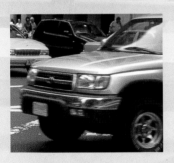

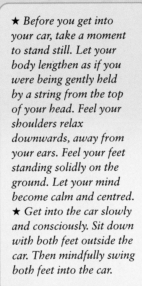

★ *Be aware of where you hold tension. In your hands? Legs? Shoulders? Check your problem areas regularly, consciously relaxing. Keep every part of your body soft and relaxed while you drive.*

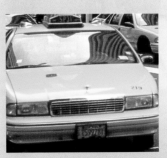

★ *When you reverse don't twist your head. Instead drop the tip of your nose to your shoulder and then turn round – it helps to lengthen the spine .*

Let it out

You're late and you're surrounded by cars driven by idiots. You can literally feel the tension rising. Fortunately your car is a sound-proof private place. Within it you can practise some of the most effective techniques for releasing tension – sound therapy – with no one being any the wiser.

SOUND STRESS BUSTERS

■ **Humming:** If you're feeling stressed, anxious, or nervous just sit quietly and hum very gently. The hum will resonate through your body. Where can you feel it? Does it change if you alter the note of the hum?

■ **Sighing:** Feeling irritable and tense? Try an elongated, noisy sigh. Deep groaning also helps to release any negative emotions. Really let go.

■ **Singing:** Tune in to cheerful music and sing along. Really belt it out. Listen to beat music when you're feeling tense – soft, soothing music can make you even more irritable!

■ **Mantras:** You don't need to say Omm or anything spiritual – simply try singing positive statements, repeating them with different tunes. For example, "I'm calm, I'm calm, I'm really calm."

These simple exercises will soon lighten your mood, and brighten your whole day.

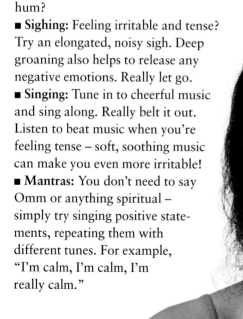

Stay alert

You've got a long drive ahead of you and you know it's going to be tough to stay focused and alert. Don't panic – just follow these simple strategies for safe long-distance driving.

★ *If you find yourself losing concentration, vary your driving speed. Keeping at one speed or relying on cruise control can be very soporific.*

★ *Do the "three-point" vision check – look just ahead of you, then into the middle distance, then to the horizon. This is good driving practice and essential when you're feeling tired.*

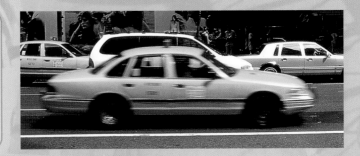

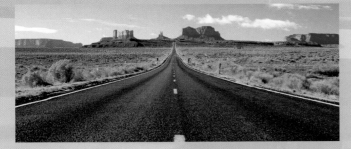

★ *Put a few drops of "wake-up" essential oils on a tissue and sniff it from time to time. The citrus scents of lemon, lime, and grapefruit are refreshing.*

★ *Use mindfulness. Be aware of everything you do and everything you see. Keep up a running commentary – "Slight tension in my neck, must relax it, a sign coming up, red car overtaking fast."*

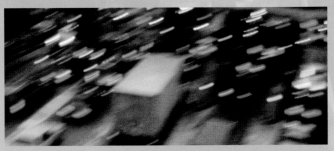

Banish road rage

When you're stuck in an unmoving traffic jam it's all too easy to let the tension levels rise. Before you know it, you're clenching your teeth and raising your voice – cursing every other driver for their stupidity. Don't allow your frustration to escalate – nip road rage in the bud with this simple exercise (though only if your car is stationary!). Use it while sitting at traffic lights or stuck in a traffic jam.

TENSION CHECKS
★ *Periodically check your shoulders and legs to make sure they are relaxed and loose.*
★ *Check your hands on the steering wheel: are you clutching it so tightly your knuckles are white? Keep as relaxed as possible.*

TENSION RELEASES
1 *Clasp your hands behind your head, so your palms are touching the back of your head.*
2 *Let the weight of your hands pull your head forward, feeling the stretch in your neck and all the way down your spine. Don't pull down; simply relax your arms and let the weight of*
your hands do all the work. Hold the position for at least 20 seconds – longer if you can.*
3 *Breathe out with a deep sigh, "A-a-a-ah."*
4 *Repeat steps 1–3 several times if possible. However, even holding it for a few seconds will release tension.*

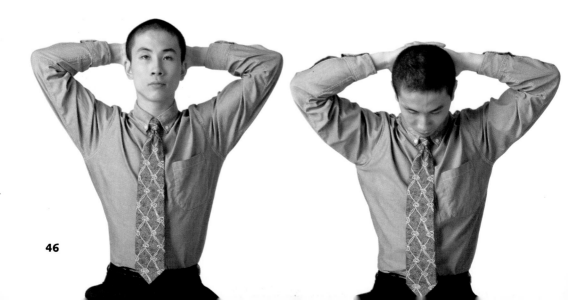

Keep your cool

Breathing exercises are one of the most effective instant ways to reduce stress and raise your energy. And the yogic breathing technique of Ujjayi, the "psychic" or "victorious" breath, is both supremely simple and remarkably powerful. Use it whenever you feel the need to "keep your cool" – your stress levels will take a dive within minutes.

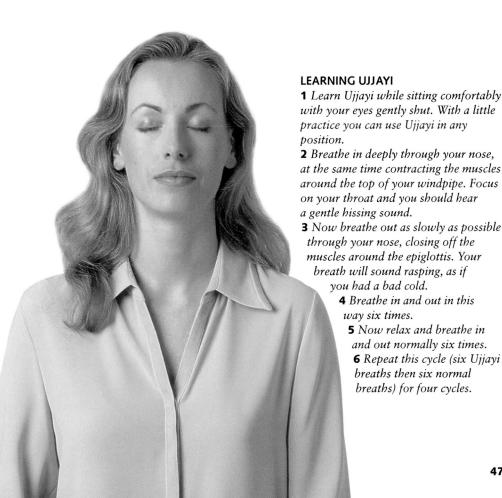

LEARNING UJJAYI

1 *Learn Ujjayi while sitting comfortably with your eyes gently shut. With a little practice you can use Ujjayi in any position.*

2 *Breathe in deeply through your nose, at the same time contracting the muscles around the top of your windpipe. Focus on your throat and you should hear a gentle hissing sound.*

3 *Now breathe out as slowly as possible through your nose, closing off the muscles around the epiglottis. Your breath will sound rasping, as if you had a bad cold.*

4 *Breathe in and out in this way six times.*

5 *Now relax and breathe in and out normally six times.*

6 *Repeat this cycle (six Ujjayi breaths then six normal breaths) for four cycles.*

Waiting in line – keeping your cool

Squashed on a crowded commuter train or waiting in line for a bus is tedious and uncomfortable. However, you can utilize this time – even if it's just a few minutes. The chi kung and yoga exercises on these pages can be performed anywhere. They help to pulse energy through the body, both calming and energizing you at the same time.

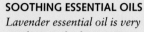

SOOTHING ESSENTIAL OILS
Lavender essential oil is very soothing and relaxing. Keep a tissue in your pocket on which you have put a couple of drops of oil. If you feel stressed or irritable, sniff it from time to time.

CHI KUNG WU CHI

1 *Stand with your feet fairly close together. Let your arms drop to your sides. If you feel safe to do so, close your eyes. Otherwise, keep them cast downwards.*
2 *Consciously work through your body, relaxing each part. Start with your head – feel your scalp relax. Let your face muscles drop, relax your jaw. Imagine even your hair is relaxing.*
3 *Crunch up your shoulders and release them. Relax your arms. Make fists and then relax your hands.*
4 *Relax your chest and your abdomen. Feel your breathing coming deeply into your abdomen, pushing it out as you breathe in. Relax your back – imagine every vertebra relaxing, your spine becoming relaxed and flexible.*
5. *Relax your hips, your thighs, let your knees become soft. Feel tension flowing down your legs and out through the soles of your feet into the ground.*

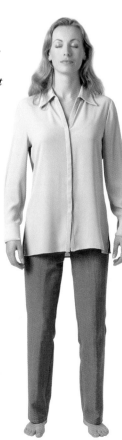

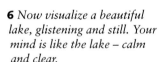

6 *Now visualize a beautiful lake, glistening and still. Your mind is like the lake – calm and clear.*
7 *Now imagine a blue sky. Clouds scud by. Any worrying thoughts are like the clouds – swiftly gone, leaving the sky pure blue and clear again.*
8 *Stay like this, relaxed and meditative, for as long as you can. When your transport arrives or you come to your destination, simply bring your awareness back to the world around you. Stamp your feet and have a good stretch.*

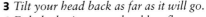

SHOULDER-SHRUGGING

1 *Sit comfortably with your arms free.*
2 *Bring your shoulders right up to your ears, shrugging as hard as you can. Intensify the tension in your body as much as possible. Breathe in as you shrug upwards.*

3 *Tilt your head back as far as it will go.*
4 *Exhale, letting your shoulders flop down and your head come up. You should feel a sense of heat in your neck and shoulders – more blood is now able to circulate through this high-tension area. Repeat as necessary.*

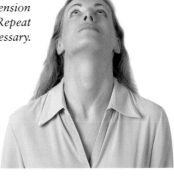

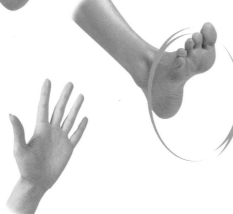

HAND AND FOOT GYMNASTICS

Repeat each step five times.
1 *Curl your toes as tight as you can and release.*
2 *Curl your entire foot down towards your heel and then stretch it upwards as far as you comfortably can.*
3 *Now circle your feet slowly clockwise and anticlockwise.*
4 *Clench your hands into fists. Then release them, opening the fingers wide.*
5 *Stretch your fingers and bend your hand back at right angles to your wrist. Then bend your hand down so your fingers point towards the floor.*
6 *Make fists again and circle clockwise and then anticlockwise.*

Balance your energy

Jin shin jyutsu is an ancient Japanese therapy that can eliminate stress and fatigue, relieve pain, and balance your emotions. The poses are simple and highly discreet – you can do jin shin anywhere – without anyone realizing.

BEAT JET LAG
This jin shin exercise helps to combat jet lag.
Hold the thumb of your left hand with the fingers of your right. When you feel a steady pulse in your thumb, release and hold the index finger of your left hand in the same way – again until you feel a pulse in the finger.
Work your way through all the fingers. Then repeat the exercise on the right hand.

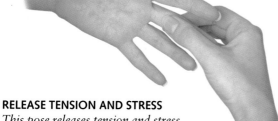

RELEASE TENSION AND STRESS
This pose releases tension and stress throughout the body. It helps to empty the body of stale and stagnant energy.
1 *Hold the middle joint of the left middle finger lightly between the right thumb and fingers.*
2 *Hold for a few minutes.*
3 *Reverse instructions for the other hand.*

CALM AND REVITALIZE YOURSELF
This pose calms the body, releasing nervous tension and stress. It also revitalizes all the organs.
1 *Hold the fourth and fifth fingers of your left hand between the thumb and fingers of your right hand, the thumb on the palm side of your left hand.*
2 *Reverse instructions for the other hand.*

Walk to success

Use the time you spend walking to coach yourself for success. Whether you have a half-hour hike or a two-minute stroll, focusing on your footsteps and giving yourself positive affirmations can make all the difference to your day.

WALK WITH MINDFULNESS

1 *Become aware of your walking. Walk a bit more slowly than normal and feel your feet touching the ground (is it hard, soft, warm, cold?). Feel your toes spreading as you walk, be aware of your knees as they bend, your hips as they swing.*

2 *Now focus your attention on your breath. Mentally say "in" as you inhale and "out" as you exhale. See if you can begin each in and each out breath exactly as one of your feet hits the ground.*

3 *Notice how many steps you take during each inhalation, and how many steps you take during each exhalation. Count each step as you walk and breathe, so that in your mind you are saying, "In two, three, four... Out two, three, four... In two, three, four" or perhaps "In two, three... Out two, three," depending on how many steps you take to each breath. You will soon find your own rhythm.*

TALK POSITIVELY
Repeat a suitable affirmation to yourself, either out loud or to yourself. Positive self-talk sends a distinct command to the subconscious – helping your affirmation become reality. Try something like "I am completely successful in everything I do" or "I am calm, focused, and in control" or "I have abundant creativity and great ideas." Repeat it over and over as you walk.

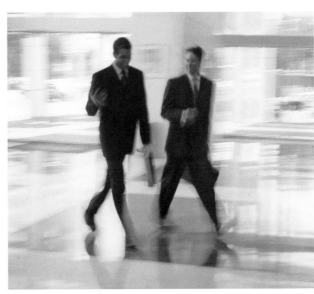

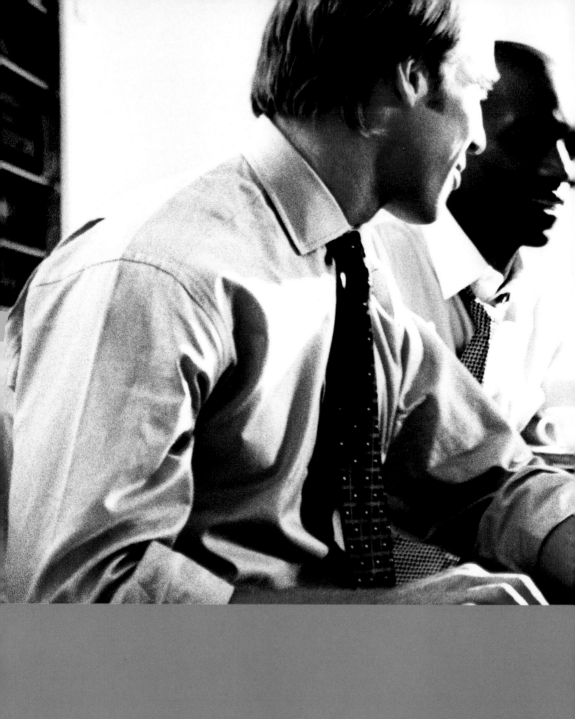

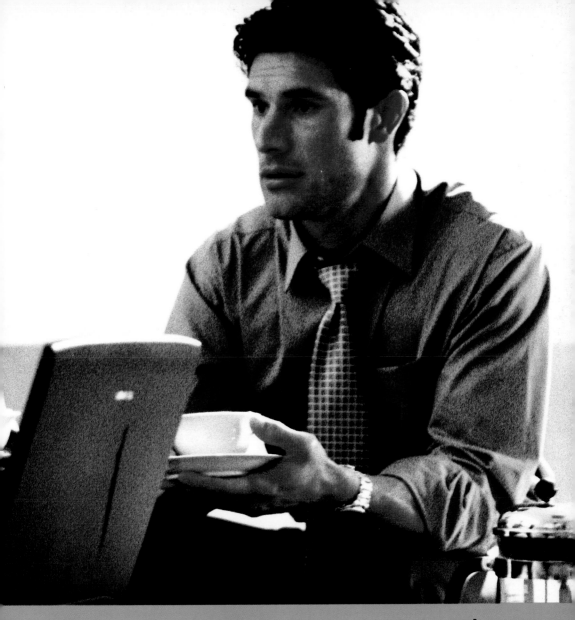

Part two: Winning at work

You've arrived at work in one piece. Now, how do you make the best of the day and come out on top?

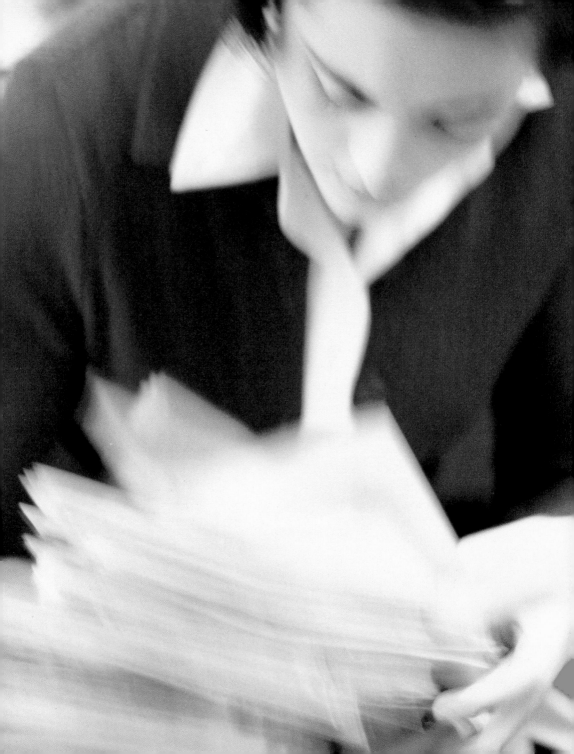

CHAPTER FOUR

Your working space

You've arrived at work. What greets you as you walk through the door? Is your place of work a calm oasis of order and tranquillity? Does it hum with a satisfying energy? Or is it a ghastly mess, full of junk and disorder?

The first step to increasing your energy and creativity, upping your productivity, and improving your mood is to make your working environment as inviting and pleasant as possible.

Nobody really wants to work in a trash can of an office. Mess makes your energy dip and clutters your mind – and searching for those all-important notes under untidy piles of papers is stressful and simply a waste of time.

So spend five minutes clearing and rearranging your working space. If you work at a desk, why not rediscover what it looks like under the acres of paper? Then you can use the Chinese art of feng shui to make your desk actually help you achieve your goals.

Whether you want an increase in salary or some extra recognition from your boss, or to improve your working relationships and get the most from your work team, how you arrange your desk can usher in a remarkable change.

We'll also take a look at how to clear the air in the office, where the overload of toxic fumes from modern furnishings, materials, and equipment can actually make people ill. Practical tips and hints show you how to banish sick office syndrome.

Neck and back strain are the banes of office life – particularly if you use a computer a lot. A short lesson on improving your sitting position, and tips for comfortable typing, take the strain out of keyboard work.

Take your working environment in hand and make it work for you. Things will change – without a shadow of a doubt.

Clear desk, clear mind: clearing clutter

A clear desk really does help you keep a clear mind. Psychologically, clutter irritates the mind. It makes us feel depressed with all the things that need doing, fixing, finishing. On an energetic level, mess pulls our energy levels down – it creates stagnant chi, or vital energy. So clear your desk and re-energize your mind.

DECLUTTERING WORK SPACES

■ Keep your desk as clear as possible. Keeping only what you are working with on it helps you to concentrate on the task in hand.

■ File papers away once you have finished working with them. Don't let them pile up on the floor.

■ When papers arrive on your desk, decide straightaway what to do with them: act on them now; file them for future use; or throw them away.

■ Keep your waste bin by your desk and open your post over it. Anything you don't need can go straight into the bin.

■ Make time to go through your filed documents and papers regularly. Throw away any that are out of date or no longer needed.

BE MORE EFFECTIVE – TOP TIPS

■ Schedule time for yourself – periods each day when you won't be interrupted. Use the time for creative work or ideas, or simply for sitting quietly and refuelling.

■ Be proactive rather than reactive. Plan what you will do and when you will do it – then stick to your plan. Treat an "appointment" with yourself like any other appointment: break it only if absolutely unavoidable.

■ Take a break every hour. Walk around for a few minutes or do a few stretches to refresh yourself and replenish your concentration.

■ Schedule your day according to your energy. Are you an early bird, or a night owl? When are you most creative, most organized? When do you feel half-asleep or on another planet? Don't plan something major for a time when you usually feel half-asleep or dreamy. Use this time to make calls, or catch up with small routine tasks.

CREATE SUCCESS: FENG SHUI YOUR DESK

Your desk is the key to success at work. Where you place your desk and what you place on it can make the difference between make and break in business – whether you are a big boss in a corporate office or self-employed in a corner of your living room. Over the next few pages we'll look at how the Chinese art of feng shui can help you arrange your desk for maximum benefit.

FOCUS YOUR MIND

★ *Keep a candle burning on your desk to focus the mind.*

★ *A few drops of bergamot or pine oil are energizing and uplifting. Rosemary oil helps concentration – but don't use it if you are pregnant or suffer from epilepsy.*

Boost your career

If you feel your career needs a general injection of life and energy, try arranging your desk this way. This is the basic template for all work spaces and will help you whatever your work and whatever your problem.

THE GOOD CAREER DESK
■ Place your desk so you sit with your back to a solid wall with a good view of the door and the window.
■ A desk lamp on one side helps focus your attention – in the top left-hand corner to improve your finances.
■ Fresh cut flowers stimulate mental activity and cleanse the atmosphere.
■ Put your telephone on the right to make the people you call more helpful. If you are left-handed, keep your address book on your right to gain a similar effect.
■ Keep essential reference books on your left-hand side – the knowledge area.
■ If your work is creative, have a rounded desk. If your work involves figures or is very precise a rectangular desk is better but ideally still with rounded corners.
■ Try to use a rectangular briefcase or handbag to make you more inclined to complete projects.
■ Your computer should be centred at the back of your desk. This area governs fame and recognition. Behind it, put something on the wall to remind you what you want to achieve – a photograph, newspaper cutting, or a collage of work goals.
■ Place something on the left-hand side to remind you of the spiritual aspect of your life. A small statue, a framed picture, or a beautiful stone.
■ Don't overload your desk with pictures of family – you will be distracted. But a couple of photos can sit in the middle and top right-hand corner.

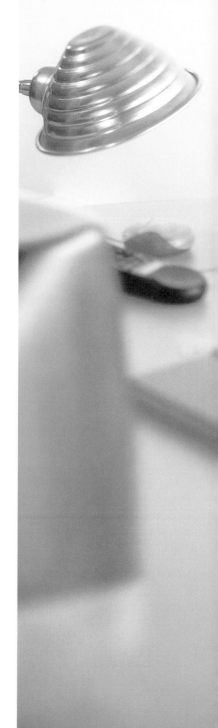

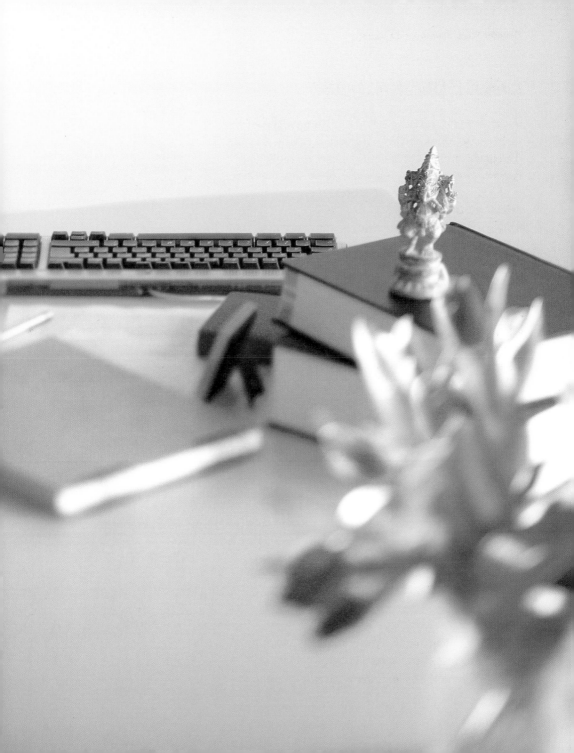

Gain recognition

Whether you want a better relationship with your boss or a nice fat raise, the art of feng shui can boost your opportunities. On the previous pages we looked at the basic template for a good desk. For more specific problems, look at these suggestions.

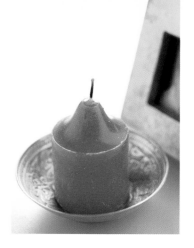

THE SALARY-RAISING DESK

To help your chances of a salary raise, you must boost the "money" area of your desk – the top left-hand corner as you sit behind it. Use as many of these "cures" as you can reasonably fit into that area.

■ Place a lamp in this corner.

■ Add a vase of flowers – ideally, four stems of red or purple flowers, which are associated with wealth in the Chinese tradition.

■ Add a crystal paperweight, a red or purple box for paper clips or spare change. Crystals are considered to boost positive energy, or chi.

■ Put your salary payment, maybe weighted down by a beautiful paperweight. Place your invoices here, too, before you send them out.

■ If you possibly can, install a fish tank with three goldfish in the left-hand corner of your desk. If not, put three Chinese coins linked with red ribbon instead.

THE CREATIVE POWERHOUSE DESK

To encourage creativity and new ideas, incorporate as many of these "cures" as you can.

■ Ensure your desk is a rounded shape or has softly rounded corners.

■ A crystal paperweight can strengthen your intuition. Place it at the centre back of your desk.

■ Keep brightly coloured fresh flowers on your desk.

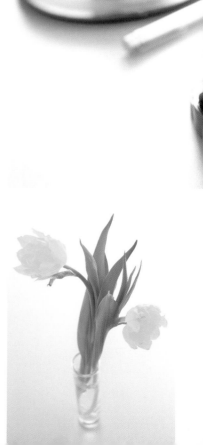

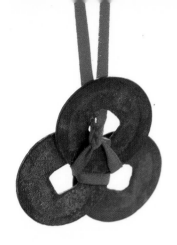

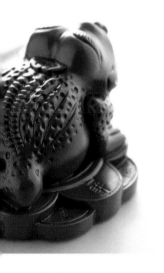

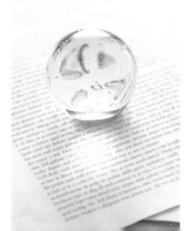

Choose desk accessories in bright, stimulating colours.
■ Place an indoor fountain near the entrance to your office or by your desk. To activate opportunities, place a three-legged toad god – a Chinese figure said to bring opportunities, luck, money, and success – on the right-hand corner of your desk.
■ Opposite you, put something that stimulates your creativity – or reminds you of your goals.

THE FAME-ENHANCING DESK

The area directly opposite you at the back of your desk is the "fame" area. If your computer occupies this space, put these enhancements and cures on or around the computer or on the wall opposite.
■ Choose something red. Or put an award or diploma here to remind you of your accomplishments.
■ A candle or crystal can make you more likely to be noticed and given recognition.
■ Make sure you have a red, purple, or yellow desk lamp to boost your fame. Add some other office accessories – desk tidies, candles, picture frames, mouse mat – in these colours, too. Strong shades stimulate mental activity and attract attention.

THE GET-ON-WITH-PEOPLE DESK

The top right-hand corner governs relationships.
■ Use yellow and the number "two" in this part of your desk – two yellow flowers in a vase perhaps.
■ Put a photograph of your work team here. Add a candle in front of it to boost the energy.
■ Move your desk lamp to this area to boost your relationship energy.

61

Combat sick office syndrome

Offices are not particularly healthy places. Some even classify as "sick" – making their inhabitants feel constantly under par and lacking in energy. Many of the materials in modern offices (paint, carpets, furniture) emit toxic fumes. If you are particularly sensitive, they could even make you physically ill. Try these strategies to minimize your risk.

SAFEGUARDING YOUR ENVIRONMENT

■ Try to work under natural light – reposition your desk by a window or use daylight bulbs. Avoid fluorescent lighting where possible.

■ Keep the office well ventilated – an open window will help discharge toxic fumes. If the weather is inclement, at the very least open the windows for just five minutes before you start work and after lunch.

■ Electrical equipment is surrounded by EMFs (electro-magnetic fields), which have been linked with insomnia, high blood pressure, anxiety, and general ill-health. So it makes sense to keep them unplugged when not in use. Position helpful plants (see opposite) by your computer, photocopier, fax, etc.

■ Use heating and air conditioning as little as possible. Think about adding another layer of clothing or installing fans to circulate cool air.

■ Make sure that any heating and air conditioning is working properly at all times – have it regularly checked and serviced.

■ Make your workplace a smoke-free zone – or have one room for smokers.

■ Install ionizers to improve the air quality. A fish-tank helps to balance the humidity of the office.

■ If you are planning to redecorate your office, use

non-toxic paints and solvents. Choose fabrics, flooring, and furniture that has not been treated with chemicals.
■ Ask your office cleaners to switch to environmentally friendly, nontoxic cleaners, detergents, etc.

THE POWER OF PLANTS

Certain plants not only make your office look good, they can also positively help your health and energy levels. Research has shown that certain species of plant can actually remove pollutants such as formaldehyde, benzene, and trichlorethylene from the air. These chemicals can be generated from carpets, MDF and fibreboard furniture, stain-protected fabrics, and paint.

SUPERPLANTS
Brighten your office with these life-enhancing plants:
★ *Golden pothos (Epipremnum aureum)*
★ *Spider plant (Chlorophytum comosum 'Vittatum')*
★ *Heartleaf philodendron (Philodendron scandens)*
★ *Monstrosus cactus (Cereus peruvianus)*
★ *Mother-in-law's tongue (Sansevieria trifasciata)*
★ *Peace lily (Spathiphyllum wallisii)*
★ *Goosefoot plant (Syngonium podophyllum)*

Ease back and neck strain

How you sit at work can have serious repercussions. If your sitting posture is bad, you can end up with chronic back and neck strain. Not only will your health suffer but your mind will never be as clear and focused as when you sit in the optimum manner. Good posture can even prevent anxiety and depression – so take a few minutes to check your seat.

Hold your head upright

HOW TO SIT
1 *Don't just throw yourself into your chair – you'll put stress on your neck, which can result in neck and back problems, or even migraines and headaches. Bend your hips and knees so that your body is balanced until you're sitting in the chair.*
2 *Think about balancing on your chair. Keep both feet firmly planted on the floor. Your weight should be equally divided between the front of your foot and your heel.*

Keep your back upright, don't hunch, and lean forwards from the waist only

Make sure your hips are slightly higher than your knees

Keep your lower legs at right angles to the floor

Put your feet flat on the floor

3 *Release your ankles, release your knees. Imagine your spine lengthening. Make sure you are sitting with equal weight on each buttock – not slumping to one side.*

4 *Is your seat high enough for you? If not, add a few telephone directories. Hunching over your desk affects breathing and all the internal organs. It's far better to lean forwards from your hip joints, so you lengthen your whole body.*

TYPING

Many of us spend our days typing on keyboards, peering at computer screens. Here's how to type with ease.

1 *Sit in an upright position, as already shown.*

2 *Stretch your arms down at your sides with your fingers facing the floor. Breathe out.*

3 *Bend your arms at the elbows and bring them up to the table, keeping your upper arms at right angles to the table, elbows slightly above desk height.*

4 *Flex your hands back from your wrists and place them softly on the keyboard. Start to type.*

5 *Check that your neck is relaxed and that you are breathing slowly and comfortably. Above all make sure your wrists stay relaxed.*

BETTER POSTURE
★ *Adjust your posture frequently when you are at work. Either consciously shift position or, ideally, get up and walk around. Setting a timer at 15 minute intervals can help to remind you.*
★ *A bulging wallet in your back trouser pocket causes you to sit unevenly with one buttock higher than the other. This twists your spine causing backache.*

Office life entails a great deal of sitting, so get your posture right and beat backache.

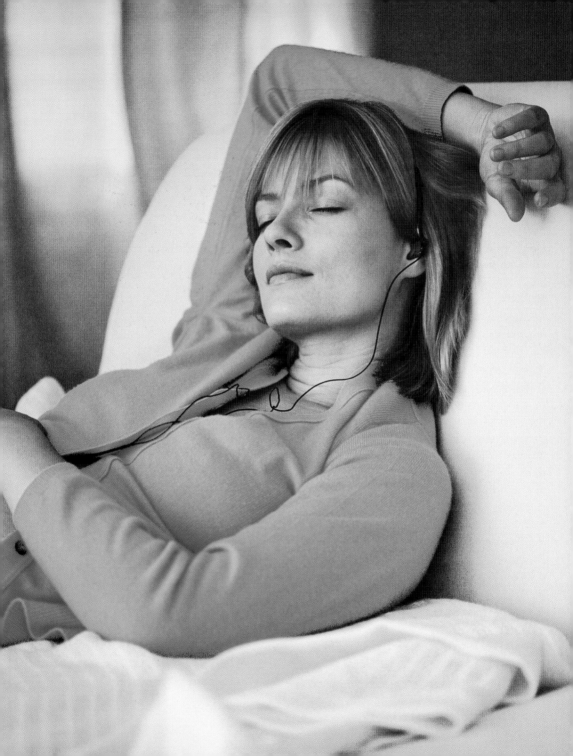

CHAPTER FIVE

Easing physical and mental stress

It's easy to get tired and stiff working in an office. Many of us spend our days staring at a computer screen or tied behind a desk for hours at a time. No wonder our bodies become stiff and tense. No wonder our eyes get sore. No wonder we find ourselves tired and yawning – before we're halfway through the morning.

If you want to get the most out of your mind, then keep your body stretched. Office yoga is the best way to do this – remarkably, you will improve your concentration while remaining relaxed and calm.

Then there is the mental strain of work to worry about. Every day offers a new challenge – a difficult meeting or a difficult colleague. People might be tetchy and unhelpful. Use the power of feng shui and NLP to help your working relationships and to steer meetings effectively. These simple techniques will teach you how to deal with difficult or downright unpleasant people.

You might well experience set-backs, disappointments, rebuffs, and refusals. Sometimes it just feels as if you're up against a brick wall and there's nowhere to turn. In cases like this it's easy to become despondent or depressed. No need. This chapter will arm you with the very latest techniques to keep your internal energy high and focused. You can combat shyness and beat off the blues; you can boost your confidence and overcome disappointment so you are ready to face the next challenge in a positive way.

So take a deep breath, relax, and let's tackle your problem head on.

Concentrate

You want to be at your best throughout your working day: alert, yet relaxed, focused, and calm. This simple shiatsu routine can help you take everything in your stride, maintaining your concentration and sailing through the day.

3 *Look up and stretch your arms, as if you were reaching for the sky, first with one hand, then the other.*

FIVE MINUTE RE-ENERGIZER
1 *Sitting at your desk, breathe in and give your shoulders a really exaggerated shrug.*

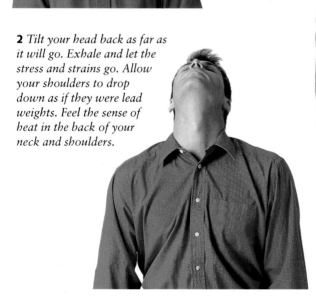

2 *Tilt your head back as far as it will go. Exhale and let the stress and strains go. Allow your shoulders to drop down as if they were lead weights. Feel the sense of heat in the back of your neck and shoulders.*

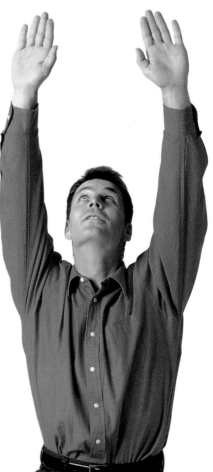

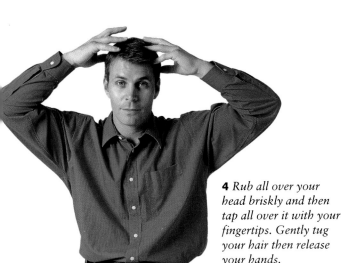

4 *Rub all over your head briskly and then tap all over it with your fingertips. Gently tug your hair then release your hands.*

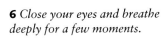

5 *Pinch all around your jawline. Then tap firmly all around your jaw with your fingertips. Clench your jaw, open your mouth wide and say (or mouth) "ahhhh."*

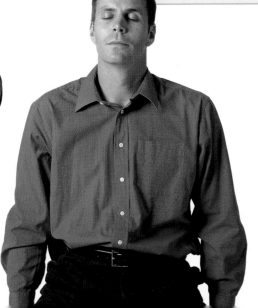

6 *Close your eyes and breathe deeply for a few moments.*

Soothe eye strain

Eyes easily become stressed and strained – particularly in air conditioned or centrally heated offices. These acupressure exercises can help you to beat the strain, or if you are feeling fuzzy-headed or tense in general.

1 Cup your hands over your eyes for a few minutes. Be gentle but firm so your eyes can still open but no light gets in.

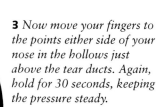

3 Now move your fingers to the points either side of your nose in the hollows just above the tear ducts. Again, hold for 30 seconds, keeping the pressure steady.

2 Use your index fingers to press the points just above the middle of your eyebrows (in line with your pupils if you were to look straight ahead). Hold with a light pressure for about 30 seconds.

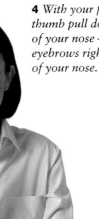

4 *With your finger and thumb pull down either side of your nose – from your eyebrows right to the end of your nose.*

5 *Now press upwards under your cheekbones with your index fingers (in about the middle of the cheekbones) and hold for 30 seconds.*

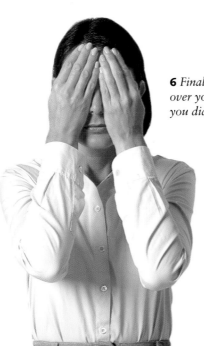

6 *Finally cup your hands over your eyes again, as you did at the beginning.*

FOCUS YOUR EYES AFAR
Working on a computer or poring over small text can cause eye strain because you focus your eyes on the near distance: take a few moments to look farther afield (out of a window or at least to the end of the office) whenever you can.

71

Instant refresher

You're trying to work but you just can't focus. These simple yoga exercises really brush away the cobwebs – they send a lightning flash of energy right through your body.

BASIC REFRESHER POSTURES

These two postures can be carried out anywhere. If you can slip off your shoes, so much the better but, if not, they will still be effective.

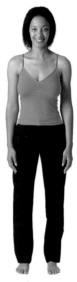
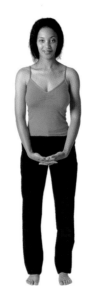
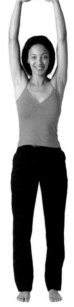
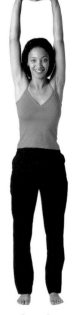

Stretch high
1 *Stand in a relaxed position, feet shoulder width apart, arms by your sides. You may like to close your eyes gently.*

2 *Clasp your hands in front of you and then slowly bring your arms above your head.*

3 *As you reach the full stretch, turn your hands so that the palms face upwards. Make sure your shoulders are relaxed. Hold this posture.*

4 *Stretch as far as is comfortable, and breathe in and out deeply through the nose several times. Slowly bring your hands back to step 1.*

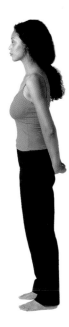

Swing low

1 *Stand with your feet shoulder width apart, knees relaxed, feet facing forwards, and eyes open so you can keep your balance.*
2 *Clasp your hands behind your back with your palms facing the floor.*

ADVANCED ENERGIZER
You need to be able to slip out of your shoes for the Swing low exercise, so if you work in a very conventional office you may need to find a quiet, out-of-the-way corner! This exercise gives your spine a really effective stretch and sends energy to every part of the body. Check with a doctor or yoga therapist if you have a bad back.

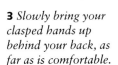

3 *Slowly bring your clasped hands up behind your back, as far as is comfortable.*

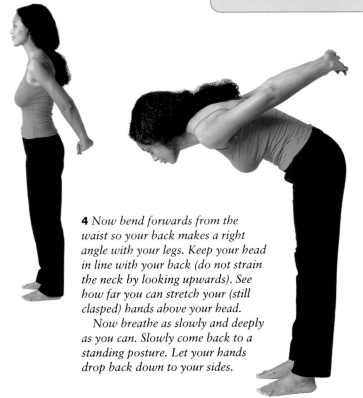

4 *Now bend forwards from the waist so your back makes a right angle with your legs. Keep your head in line with your back (do not strain the neck by looking upwards). See how far you can stretch your (still clasped) hands above your head.*

Now breathe as slowly and deeply as you can. Slowly come back to a standing posture. Let your hands drop back down to your sides.

You can do it

The key to success at work (and anywhere else) is self-confidence. If you believe in yourself, you can achieve almost anything. But sometimes that is easier said than done. When you feel a bit overwhelmed or lacking in nerve, try these simple confidence-boosters.

POWER POSTURE

How you hold yourself can have an immediate and powerful effect on your mood. If you look confident, you will actually become more confident.
1 Stand or sit tall and upright. Imagine that the top of your head is attached to the ceiling with a piece of string.
2 Let your shoulders relax downwards. Mentally run through your body and make sure you are not holding tension in the classic places – face, jaw, neck, shoulders, buttocks, thighs, hands.

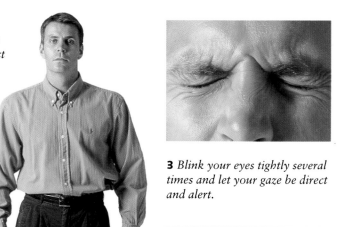

> **CAUTION**
> **Do not** *hold this posture for a long period if you have high blood pressure, heart disease, or if you are pregnant or menstruating.*

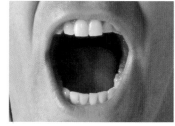

3 Blink your eyes tightly several times and let your gaze be direct and alert.

4 Yawn widely to stretch your jaw. Smile. Repeat silently to yourself a positive affirmation, e.g. "I am brimming with self-confidence; everything works for me" or "I now choose success in everything I do."

STAND TALL AS A MOUNTAIN

This Mountain posture is adapted from chi kung. It's very simple but has a powerful effect on your mood. It invigorates your whole body and mind while making you feel grounded and powerful. Find a quiet spot to try this – or pretend you're just having a good stretch!

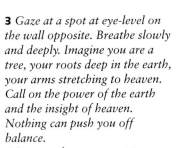

1 *Stand in the basic chi kung starting posture (page 16). Bring your fingers together and point them straight down to the ground.*

2 *Raise your arms slowly from step 1, keeping them stretched. Extend your arms out to the side. As you reach shoulder height, turn the palms upwards and continue to lift your arms until they are pointing directly upwards (parallel to your ears). Keep your shoulders relaxed.*

3 *Gaze at a spot at eye-level on the wall opposite. Breathe slowly and deeply. Imagine you are a tree, your roots deep in the earth, your arms stretching to heaven. Call on the power of the earth and the insight of heaven. Nothing can push you off balance.*
4 *Reverse the movement to release the posture: bring your arms back to shoulder height; turn your palms down; relax your arms by your sides. Stand quietly for a moment. Feel the energy in your body.*

75

Combat shyness

Shyness can be a nightmare – particularly in the workplace. First of all remember that everyone is shy sometimes – you're not alone. Then try this NLP technique at home; it taps into your subconscious mind to find the answer to your shyness problem.

NEGOTIATE WITH YOUR BODY

1 Sit or lie down in a comfortable position. Close your eyes, breathe deeply and allow yourself to relax.
2 Become aware of your body. Now let one part of it come to mind – whichever part appears first. You will be communicating directly with this body part.
3 Ask who or what is there. It could be a shape, a creature, or a person. It might be a large black blob, a snake, your mother, or an early teacher, for example. Ask it what its intention is. What purpose does it have in this part of your body? It might be trying to protect you; to shield you from embarrassment, to stop you making a fool of yourself.
4 Once it has given its reply, ask it if it wouldn't rather do something else? Whether it would rather have its freedom? Listen for its answer.
5 If it says "yes" thank it for having been there and release it. You may want to look deeply at it – see what

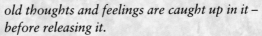

*old thoughts and feelings are caught up in it –
before releasing it.*
6 *If it says "no" you may not be ready to give up
this part. Look deeply into it and see what limiting
self-beliefs and old attitudes are caught up in it.
Maybe it would be willing to change in some
constructive way. Perform this exercise frequently
until you have got to the bottom of the problem
and can allow whatever controls that part of
your body to let go and be released.*

BACH FLOWER REMEDIES

*Simply add one or two drops of a remedy to a glass
of water and sip it throughout the day whenever
you feel the need. Choose the remedy that most
closely matches your symptoms. Remember, you
can combine the remedies but don't use more
than five together.*

★ ***Agrimony:*** *you seem cheerful and on top
of things but are secretly worried, fearful,
and lacking in confidence.*

★ ***Mimulus:*** *you're fearful and lack courage.
You're scared of everyday things and are very timid.*

★ ***Larch:*** *you lack confidence in your abilities;
you are afraid of failure and so don't try.*

★ ***Elm:*** *you're usually confident but sometimes find
responsibility too much and become despondent.*

★ ***Hornbeam:*** *you don't feel you have enough
strength for the day ahead, the task in hand. You
put things off until tomorrow.*

★ ***Scleranthus:*** *you're indecisive and hesitating
all the time.*

Diffuse arguments

Arguments and disagreements happen. They're only natural. But you can stop them becoming unpleasant and creating tension in the office with this visualization technique. As soon as you feel a difficult situation arising say "let's have a five minute break and come back to this." Use this time to go somewhere quiet and use this technique.

■ Sit or lie down and breathe calmly and deeply for a few minutes.

■ Write down the reasons for your argument. You can pour out all your resentment and any feelings of anger.

■ Can you see the other person's point of view? If not, take two chairs. Sit on one and imagine the other person is sitting on the other chair. Tell them exactly why you were so angry. Now swap chairs and imagine you are the other person. What are their reasons for feeling angry? Allow yourself to slip into their shoes and express their grievances. You can swap chairs like this for as long as it takes to understand both sides of the question. Try to accept that there are two sides to every argument.

■ Even if you still disagree with the other person at the end of this time, recognize that they have a right to their opinion. If it's safe to do so, burn the piece of paper containing your grievances.

■ Visualize love and forgiveness shooting out from your heart chakra (energy centre) to their's. Imagine it as a beautiful pink-gold colour.

■ Return to the person with whom you're arguing and smile genuinely at them. Suggest you continue over a warm drink or even a glass of wine after work. You should find the situation has totally changed.

EXTRA HELP

If you can't get away from your workplace for even five minutes, then try these instant tension-busters for extra help. The first is an aromatherapy essential oil and the second is a flower remedy:

★ *Put two drops of pine essential oil on a tissue and breathe in the scent. Pine helps foster forgiveness and fair-mindedness; the two drops represent the two of you involved in the argument. Avoid pine essential oil if you are suffering from high blood pressure.*

★ *Put two drops of Beech flower remedy under your tongue. Beech helps resolve bitterness and anger; it stops you being over-critical. If your partner in argument will take some too, so much the better.*

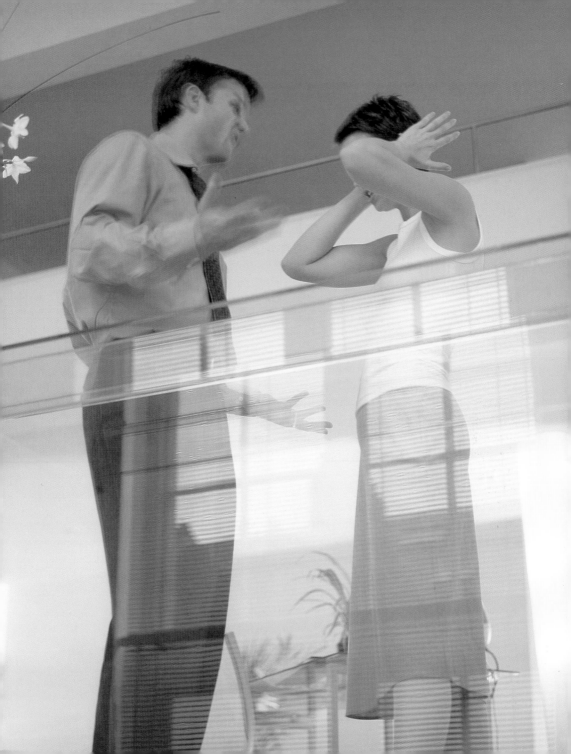

Power meetings

When you've got an important or tough meeting ahead of you, maximize your position by using a secret tactic: feng shui. The Chinese art of placement allows you to come out on top by the most subtle means.

THE BUSINESS MEETING OR LUNCH

Whether you are meeting important clients or colleagues, it's essential you feel as comfortable as possible and exude a sense of calm confidence.

■ Choose a chair whose back is reasonably close to a wall. Ideally, you will be able to see the door (but not be in a direct line with it). Make sure you don't have your back to a door or window.

■ Now invite the more senior of your guests to sit opposite you. This shows respect.

■ The more junior person should sit on your left, which is good for harmonious discussions.

■ Other people can take the remaining places.

■ If possible, choose a round table, which signifies that business will go profitably, smoothly, efficiently, and fairly quickly.

■ A round glass or paperweight makes a good centrepiece, perhaps arranged with flowers or candles.

■ Place three coins under the glass paperweight and a mirror under the coins. The three coins represent growth and movement connected to money and the glass paperweight strengthens the intuition of all concerned and creates a more harmonious settlement.

■ Use the power of colour to help your meeting. Choose folders and paperclips in the appropriate colour to boost your meeting. Red for publicity; yellow for dealing with important people; purple for finance; green or blue for creativity and growth.

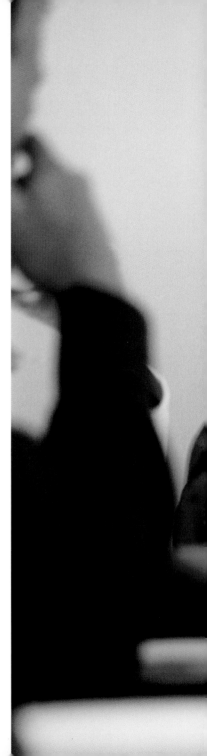

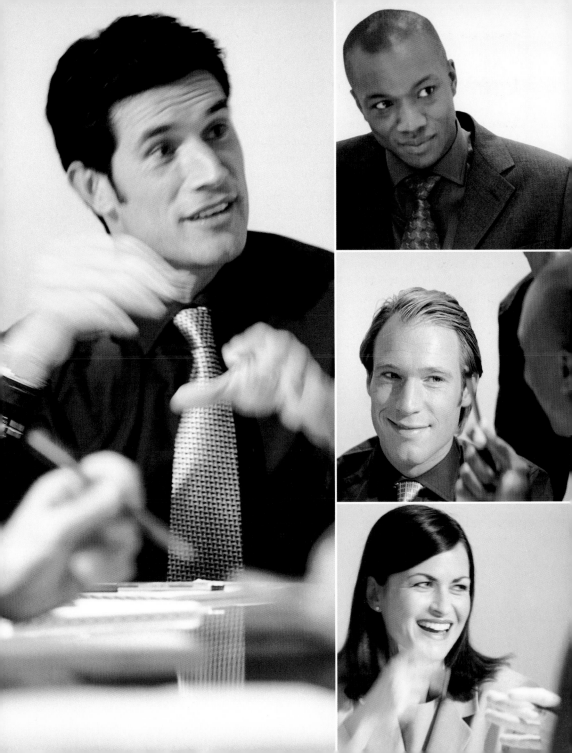

Creating rapport

Some people we like immediately; others seem to be on another planet completely. It's an energy thing – some people are literally on the same energetic wavelength as we are. In our private lives we can pick our friends; yet at work we have to get on with quite difficult people. Here's how, using NLP strategies.

BODY LANGUAGE

NLP teaches you how to gain rapport with someone quickly and easily, by matching their body language.
■ Become aware of the other person. Are they sitting or standing? In a relaxed or formal posture? Do they hold

Eye contact is fundamental to creating rapport. Try to reach a common level but don't let it interfere with communication.

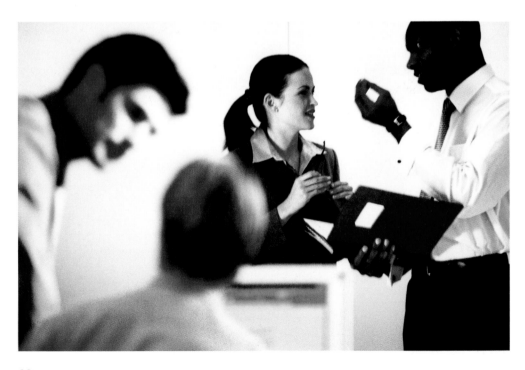

their head up erect? Or sway, or keep their head tilted to one side? Or have a rounded posture with their head down? Subtly echo their stance – without its looking as though you are mimicking them.

■ Let the other person set the agenda for personal space. If they move in closer, don't move away. Equally, don't move in on them.

■ How much eye contact do they make? Try to match it.

■ Become aware of how they breathe. Is it high in the chest, mid-range, or low down in the abdomen? If you can, shift your breathing to match theirs.

■ How do they speak? Fast or slow? High pitched, or low and soft, or melodic with natural rhythm. Don't parody their speech but if you find yours is wildly out of sync adjust it accordingly.

VERBAL LANGUAGE

Listen to the language they use. Most people have one favourite sense they rely on when reacting to the world: visual, audio or kinesthetic (feeling). You can tell a person's dominant sense by the words and phrases they use.

■ Visual: "I see what you mean." "I get the picture." "My point of view…" "I take a dim view of…"

■ Auditory: "I hear what you're saying." "We're on the same wavelength." "Speak your mind!" "What do you say to…."

■ Kinesthetic: "I get the feeling that…" "You put your finger on it." "Hold on a moment!" "Let's get to grips with this."

You can then "pace" the person, using words and phrases from "their" language. This puts them at ease and makes them feel you're on the same wavelength.

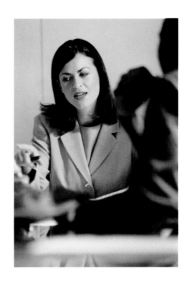

Personal space is important. Try to let the other person set the agenda but don't let them dominate your space.

Banish the blues

Almost everyone feels down from time to time. You want to run away and hide but, instead, you have to crack on with the day. Homeopathy, aromatherapy, and flower essences can help banish the black dog.

BACH FLOWER REMEDIES

These remedies, developed by Dr Edward Bach in the 1930s, are like homeopathic remedies. They are made from the flowers of wild plants. Put two drops in a glass of water and sip it four times a day or as needed.

REMEDY	SYMPTOMS
MUSTARD	*When you're depressed for no apparent reason – like a passing cloud.*
WHITE CHESTNUT	*When you have worrying thoughts that go round and round in your mind, giving no peace.*
ELM	*If you're usually confident but feel the pressure of work just too much to cope with and then feel despairing and despondent.*
GORSE	*You are pessimistic and see only negative outcomes. You've lost hope.*
WILD ROSE	*You are unmotivated and resigned. You are apathetic and not interested in change.*
WILLOW	*You dwell on your own misfortunes and negativity. You tend to be resentful and bitter, finding it hard to forgive and forget.*
GENTIAN	*You are a pessimist and full of self-doubt. Depression and melancholia are brought on by a set-back or difficulty.*

AROMATHERAPY

Try putting a few drops of one of the following oils on a tissue and sniffing it. If possible, use one of these oils in a diffuser or burner or put a couple of drops on a shower mitt and rub yourself with it in the bath or shower – but avoid the face and any sensitive areas.

REMEDY	SYMPTOMS
CEDARWOOD	*Stimulates the mind and is invigorating. Can help release anxiety or fear and lift depression. Avoid in pregnancy.*
LIME	*Refreshing and uplifting – ideal when you're tired, apathetic, anxious, and depressed. Avoid if skin is sensitive.*
NEROLI	*Re-energizing – it gives confidence and balances the emotions. Ideal if you have had a bad shock or are feeling panicky, tense, or depressed.*
BERGAMOT	*Soothing for the nerves and uplifting for the mind. Balances energies and is ideal if you're stressed, anxious, depressed, or sad.*

HOMEOPATHY

The following are the three classic homeopathic remedies for depression. Choose the remedy that most closely seems to match your symptoms. Try taking your remedy, usually as a pill, in the 30th potency (30c). If you find you cannot come through the depression, visit your doctor.

AURUM	*You are basically an idealist but feel totally worthless, disgusted with your self and your life. You fear failure. You are oversensitive to noise and excitement.*
NATRUM MURIATICUM (NAT MUR)	*You are sad but can't weep. You dwell on past griefs. You don't like company but equally don't want to be alone. You are a dignified person and don't want consolation.*
SEPIA	*You feel careworn, pathetic, weepy, overwhelmed, irritable, easily offended. You get anxious towards evening.*

Overcome disappointment

Life doesn't always go according to plan. We all have to face disappointment, rejection, and set-backs from time to time. The following visualization is a form of self-hypnosis that can help you overcome disappointment, put things into a better perspective, and restore your energy and equilibrium.

1 Find somewhere quiet where you won't be disturbed. Sit or lie down in a comfortable position. Close your eyes.

2 Become aware of your breathing. Gradually let it become deeper and more relaxed. As you breathe in, be aware of your abdomen rising; as you breathe out, take note of it falling. It is important to concentrate on your breathing rather than on your problem.

3 Now imagine you are in a large open space. In front of you stands a large wheel, like a Ferris wheel in a fairground. Watch carefully as the wheel goes round and round until it gradually comes to a stop. There's an illusion, since it seems to go backwards yet continues going forwards. Look at the people inside the wheel as they ascend into the air and then descend, coming close to the ground.

4 Follow the wheel with your eyes for a few minutes, turning your head as the wheel turns. As it goes upwards say to yourself, "I'm going up" and when it comes down, "I'm going down." Let yourself feel calm, detached, and serene – it doesn't really matter whether you go down, you will always go up again. Feel the peace within you.

5 Choose a positive affirmation – one that works for

you – to back up this feeling. Something along the lines of "I am calm, I am calm" or "Whether I go upwards or downwards, it all works for the best" or "Up and down, calm and serene." Repeat this phrase to yourself, either silently or out loud, as you follow the movement of the wheel.

6 Now stop turning your head. Affirm to yourself that you will not let yourself become down and depressed by failure any more. Remind yourself that every disappointment, every rejection, and every set-back is just a down turn of the wheel. Nobody who is truly successful has made it without set-backs. The same goes for you – this is just a glitch.

7 Remind yourself of your goals and repeat your commitment to getting there. Open your eyes, stand up, stretch, and stamp your feet to ground yourself. Make yourself a drink and maybe a snack to come back to full waking reality. Be assured your luck *will* change.

NOTE: If you know you are the sort of person who handles disappointments and set-backs badly, then repeat this visualization regularly for the best possible results. Otherwise, you need only turn to it when you are feeling down.

Change your mood with music

Want to shift your mood quickly? Try music therapy –
a powerful but simple technique that can swiftly shift
negative moods (if you can, try it in the workplace). It
can also help you beat stress and boost energy levels.

ENTRAINMENT
Music therapy works by entrainment – a simple but
powerful technique. You merge with, or synchronize
to, the pulse of the music. First match your current
mood with music that perpetuates that mood. Then,
gradually, you can shift your mood by altering the
selection of music.

MAKING AN ENTRAINMENT TAPE
You can use entrainment to alter virtually any mood.
You will need a tape recorder and a tape of 30 to 45
minutes per side.

■ Choose two or three pieces of music that match your
present mood (e.g. low confidence, blues, anxiety) and
record them at the beginning of the tape. So, if you're
down, the music will probably be gloomy or
lugubrious; if you're anxious, it might be
rasping or very fast tempo.

■ Now select three or four musical pieces that fall
somewhere between your present mood and the state
you want to achieve (e.g. confident, uplifted, calm).
So, in other words, less gloomy or anxious but still
quite moderated. Start with the most subdued and
work to the most cheery.

■ Complete your tape's musical sequence with three
or four musical pieces that match your desired state as
closely as possible. So, if you're looking for an uplifted
mood, you might choose something like the

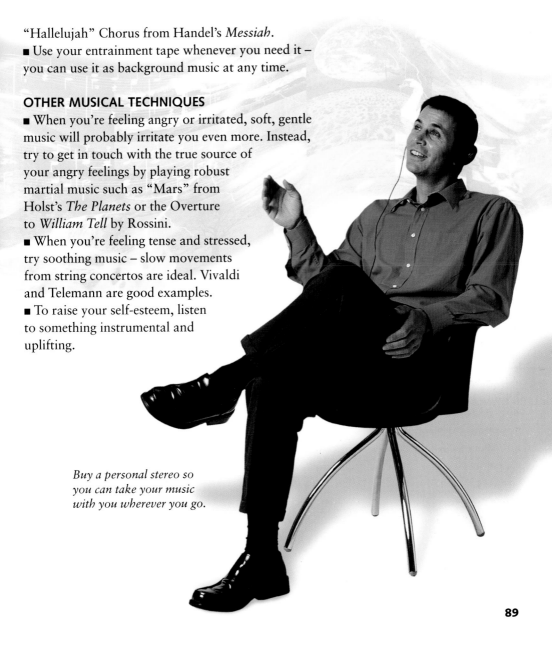

"Hallelujah" Chorus from Handel's *Messiah*.
■ Use your entrainment tape whenever you need it –
you can use it as background music at any time.

OTHER MUSICAL TECHNIQUES
■ When you're feeling angry or irritated, soft, gentle
music will probably irritate you even more. Instead,
try to get in touch with the true source of
your angry feelings by playing robust
martial music such as "Mars" from
Holst's *The Planets* or the Overture
to *William Tell* by Rossini.
■ When you're feeling tense and stressed,
try soothing music – slow movements
from string concertos are ideal. Vivaldi
and Telemann are good examples.
■ To raise your self-esteem, listen
to something instrumental and
uplifting.

Buy a personal stereo so
you can take your music
with you wherever you go.

89

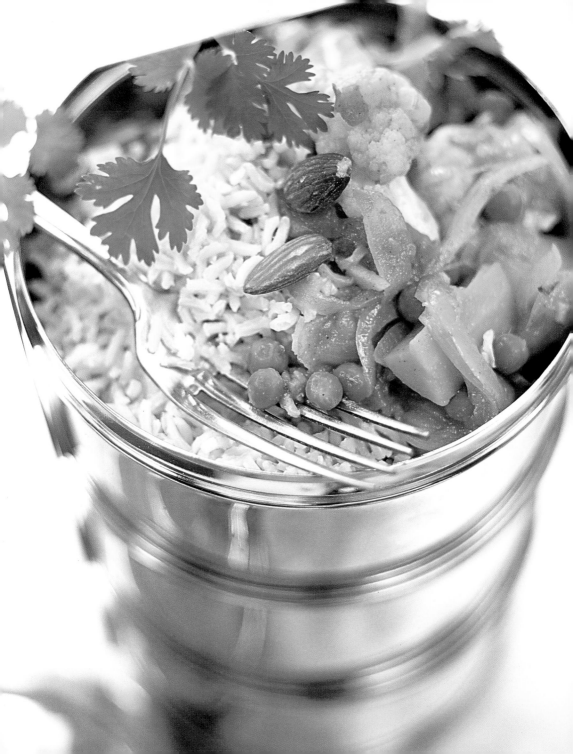

CHAPTER SIX

Have a break

Lunch-time. The crucial mid-point of the day. Time to refuel and revitalize yourself. If you've had a good morning, it can be easy to let the afternoon slide away: take a few minutes to refresh and re-energize yourself. If, on the other hand, the morning has been pretty hideous, all is not lost. Imagine the day is two completely separate segments: put the morning behind you and focus on the new half of the day ahead.

Anything is possible with the right attitude. Lunch-time is the perfect chance to snatch five minutes for meditation to release the tensions of the morning or for a quick yoga routine to shake out the stresses and boost your energy for the afternoon. If you're feeling hot or irritable, some cooling, calming breathwork will work wonders.

Traditional Chinese chi kung exercises that you can do at your desk will balance your energies and stimulate your whole system. And if you can find somewhere quiet, why not try using the power of sound to put you straight back in control of your day?

You also need to make time for a healthy lunch or a wholesome snack. It isn't like breakfast, when you really need something decent – for lunch, people vary in their needs and a full lunch is not always practical. The food you choose is crucially important. Eat the wrong foods, and you will feel sluggish all afternoon. Eat the optimum lunch, and you will feel bright, alert, and full of energy.

Your food choices can even boost your memory or your mental performance. Business lunches needn't leave you overfull and sleepy – choose wisely and you will be perfectly prepared to get the afternoon going with a bang.

LEFT: See Appendix (pages 152–153) for Vegetable curry with wild rice recipe   **91**

Refuel, revitalize

Can the foods you eat shift your mood as well as assuage your hunger? The latest research reveals you could do anything from beating depression to boosting your memory simply by choosing the right food.

EAT FOR ENERGY

To boost your energy levels choose foods from:
protein-rich wonder-foods: seafood – shrimp, fish, scallops, mussels (not for pregnant women); turkey breast; nonfat milk; lowfat or nonfat yogurt.
foods containing boron: fruit (apples, pears, peaches, grapes); nuts; broccoli; legumes.

ENHANCE YOUR MEMORY

To boost your memory choose foods from:
foods high in thiamin: wheatgerm, bran, nuts, or fortified cereals.
foods containing riboflavin: almonds, fortified cereals, milk, or liver (not for pregnant women).
foods containing carotene: dark green, leafy vegetables, orange fruits, or vegetables.
foods rich in zinc: seafood (not for pregnant women), legumes, cereals, or wholegrains.

BUSINESS LUNCHES

A good menu to enhance your mental performance and alertness: salad made from salad greens, tomato, feta cheese, baked tofu, and fat-free dressing; wholegrain roll; wholemeal pasta with prawns and broccoli; fruit salad; peach smoothie made with nonfat yogurt and milk.

See Appendix (pages 152-153) for Seafood stir-fry recipe.

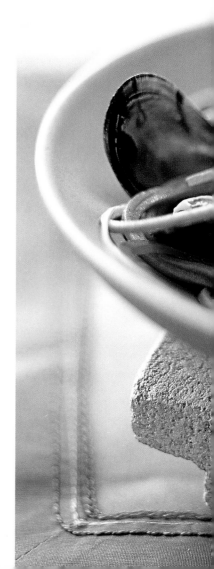

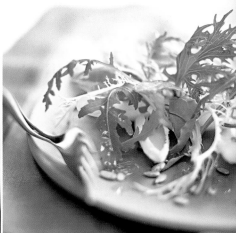

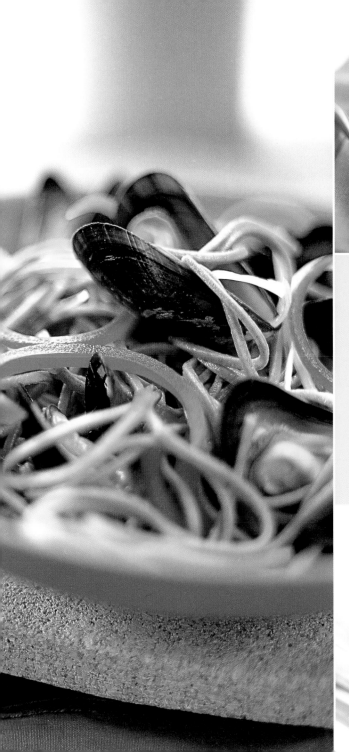

WHAT TO AVOID
★ *Saturated animal fat (red meat, bacon, sausages, etc.)*
★ *Butter*
★ *Alcohol*
★ *Caffeine (including chocolate and sodas)*
★ *Any processed food*
★ *Artificial sweeteners that are often found in diet foods*
★ *Food with additives, colourings, or preservatives*

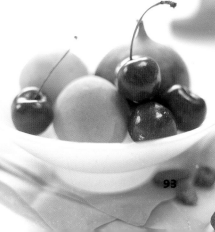

Recharge your batteries

Palming meditation gives your whole system a mini-break – any time, anywhere. Your heartbeat will slow down, your breathing will become steady and relaxed. You will feel tension dropping from your body.

PALMING MEDITATION

1 *Sit with your elbows on a desk and put your face in your hands, cupping your palms over your eyes. Don't press – your touch should be light and gentle.*
2 *Relax your shoulders and sink into the soothing darkness.*
3 *As you sit quietly, feel the gentle warmth of your hands permeating every cell of your eyes. The vital energy transmitted through your palms fills your eyes with energy, wisdom, and renewed clarity. Affirm to yourself that you will see clearly and truthfully this afternoon.*
4 *Now visualize your third eye in the centre of your forehead (it governs intuition and psychic awareness). Feel that area becoming energized. Affirm to yourself that you will call on your intuition throughout the rest of the day – you will make the right choices, the right decisions.*
5 *Rest quietly like this for as long as possible.*
6 *Come back to waking reality. Stamp your feet to re-establish contact with the everyday world.*

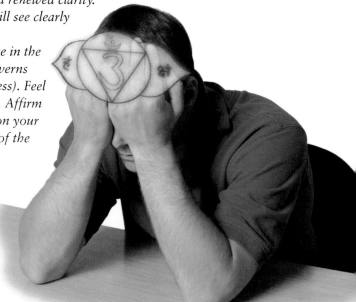

Cool down

The yogic cooling breath is very soothing and relaxing. It is also ideal for hot summer days when you feel overheated and irritable. It brings in cooling air, soothing the overheated energy of the body.

COOLING BREATH

1 *Sit down in a comfortable position. Place your hands gently on your knees. Close your eyes and become aware of your natural breathing pattern.*
2 *Curl up your tongue into a tube, letting the tip protrude slightly out of your lips. If you cannot do this, just keep your mouth slightly open and allow the air to come in over your tongue.*
3 *Breathe in slowly and deeply through the gap in your tongue. You will feel a rush of cool air on your tongue.*
4 *Now breathe out in the same way, slowly and deeply. Continue like this for a few minutes, or as long as you feel comfortable. You should notice a cooling effect down your spine and spreading out through your entire body.*
5 *Return to normal breathing, focusing on your natural breath. Once again, become aware of your surroundings.*
6 *Cast your gaze downwards then slowly open your eyes. Focus on how you feel: sit still for a few moments and feel how the energy in your body has shifted.*

Don't worry if you are unable to to curl your tongue properly – you will find the excerise just as effective.

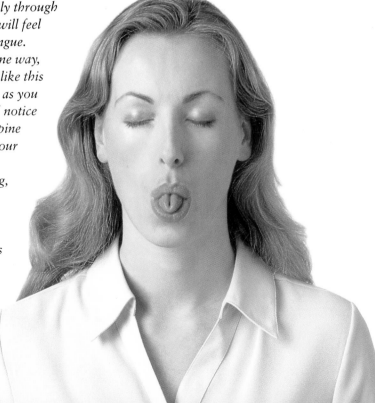

Rebalance body and mind

Halfway through the day you need something to boost your energy levels and shake out the stresses of the morning. This series of yoga moves will stretch out your body and reduce stiffness; they will improve your digestion and boost the energy throughout your system. Perform this series of exercises before you eat your lunch.

> **CAUTION**
> *Check with your doctor before trying this series of moves if you are pregnant, if you have high blood pressure or heart disease, or back or joint problems.*

A REFRESHING SHOWER OF ENERGY
Once you are familiar with this routine, repeat it several times – either slowly or dynamically, according to your mood.

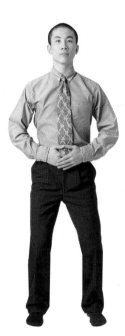

1 *Start in the basic standing posture (see chi kung, page 16). Place your hands softly across your stomach – just below your navel – and inhale deeply through your nose.*

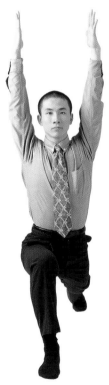

2 *Exhale through your mouth with an explosive "ha!" sound. At the same time, lunge your right leg forwards. Lift your arms up with the palms facing each other (warrior pose). Make sure your knee is directly over your ankle and you are looking straight ahead. Inhale through your nose as you lunge back to the starting position (step 1). Repeat on your left side.*

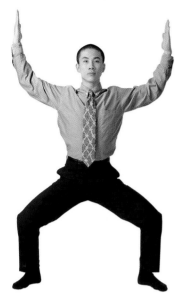

3 *Exhale through the mouth saying "ha!" as you move your right foot out to the right, bending both legs into a squat. At the same time bring your arms up and out at shoulder level with your hands pointing upwards, palms facing each other. Inhale through your nose as you lunge back to starting position (step 1). Repeat, starting with your left foot.*

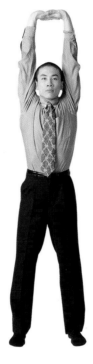

4 *Clasp your hands in front of your stomach and inhale as you bring them up over your head, turning your palms out so that they face upwards.*
Exhale, bend your knees, and lower your arms to your stomach. Repeat three or four times.

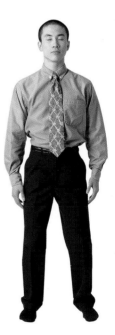

5 *Straighten your knees and come back to the basic standing posture (step 1), hands by your sides. Close your eyes and feel your energy.*

Let go of a bad morning

You've had a rough morning and are dreading the afternoon ahead. You desperately need to let go of the past few hours and rebalance your energy in order to cope with the remaining part of your working day. Tapping and breathing are simple ways to stimulate and balance your energy.

THE THREE TAPS

The Chinese system of chi kung teaches that rhythmically tapping various parts of the body creates a vibrational wave deep into the tissues, stimulating blood circulation and balancing your entire energy flow. These are the classic "Three Taps."

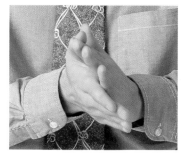

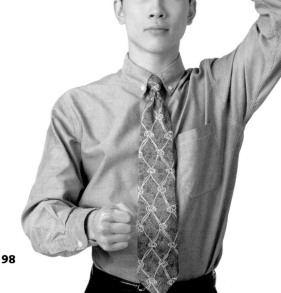

THE HEAD AND NECK TAP
1 *Rub your palms briskly together until they are warm.*
2 *Make fists but with your thumbs clenched against the outside of your index fingers.*

3 *Using your knuckles and the bottom of your fist, tap vigorously around the back of your neck and head. Go up both sides of your spine, moving from the top of the shoulders up the neck to the base of the skull, then over the skull to the top of the forehead and back down the neck again. Keep to the mid-line but extend all over your head.*

THE KIDNEYS AND ADRENAL TAP

Use the back of your fists to gently tap the left and right kidneys alternately, from top to bottom. You'll find the kidneys just above your waist at the back of the abdomen on either side of your spine. Tap each area for around two minutes.

THE THYMUS TAP

Using the middle row of the knuckles of one hand, tap the centre of your chest rhythmically. The beat is one heavy tap followed by two lighter taps (ONE, two, three, ONE, two, three). Tap for around two minutes.

99

Gain total control – sound meditation

Is there somewhere at work you can go where you won't be disturbed? If so, you have the perfect chance to rebalance your energy in your lunch hour. Sound is a profound healer, and intoning various sounds can bring all the seven chakras, or energy centres, of your body into optimum balance.

INTONING THE CHAKRAS

1 *Sit down in a comfortable position and gently close your eyes. Spend a few moments following your breath, just being aware.*
2 *Take a deep breath and focus your attention on the root chakra, at the bottom of the spine. Imagine the colour red and make a very deep "uhhh" sound, feeling the sound vibrate around the base of your spine and around your genital region, grounding you and making you stable.*
3 *Continue moving up the chakras – see chart opposite for the sounds to make, the colours to visualize, the feelings to imagine. As you start, the sounds are deep; as you move upwards, the sounds become progressively higher in tone.*
4 *Finally, move to the crown chakra, a glowing sphere of golden white at the top of your head. The sound here is a very high "eee" (as in me or she) – as high as you can go. As you intone this sound, visualize yourself connecting to your highest self and to your sense of the spiritual. Then visualize all the chakras linking up as the energy of this sound shoots down through your body, balancing as it descends.*
5 *Sit quietly for a few moments, returning to normality. Stamp your feet and open your eyes. Eat something after this exercise to ground you completely.*

THE SEVEN CHAKRAS
The chakras are centres of vital energy in your body. There are seven of them (see right), from the root chakra at the base of the spine to the crown chakra just above the head. When all the chakras vibrate in balance, we enjoy perfect health and wellbeing.

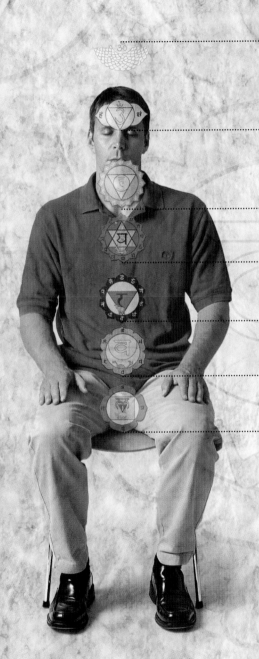

Crown chakra: *just above head. Sound:* *"eee' (as in me). Colour: golden white. Feeling: connecting to the higher self and the spiritual.*

Third eye: *middle of the brow. Sound: "ay" (as in day). Colour: indigo. Feeling: insight; knowledge; intuition.*

Throat chakra: *throat. Sound: "eye". Colour: blue. Feeling: calmness; clear communication.*

Heart chakra: *heart. Sound: "ah" (as in father). Colour: green. Feeling: compassion; love for yourself and others.*

Solar plexus chakra: *between breastbone and navel. Sound: "oh" (as in mow). Colour: yellow. Feeling: personal power.*

Sacral chakra: *genitals. Sound: "ooooo". Colour: orange. Feeling: self-worth; positivity.*

Root chakra: *at base of spine. Sound: "uhhh". Colour: red. Feeling: grounded and stable.*

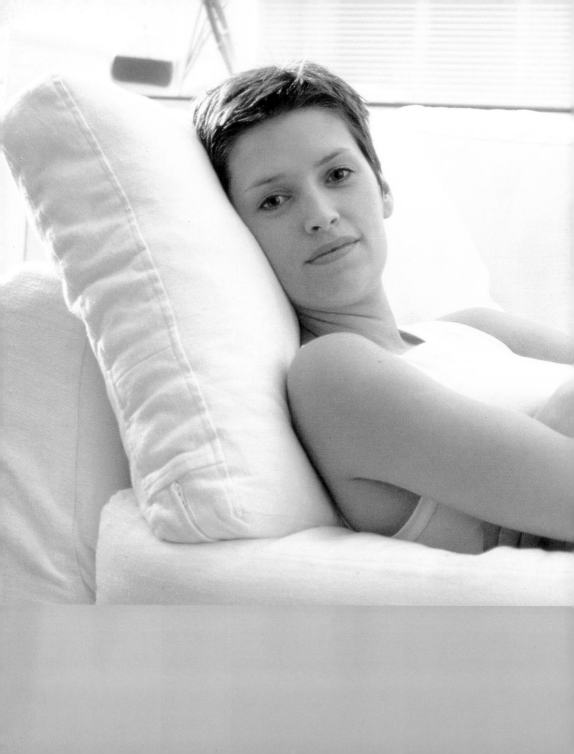

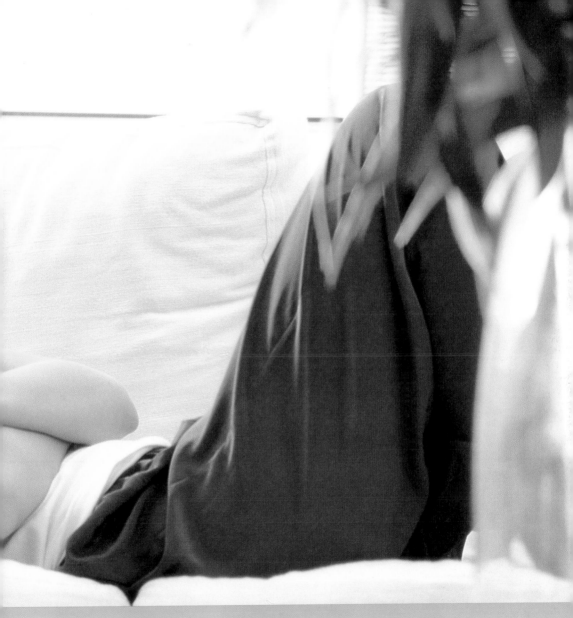

Part three: After work

Free from work, evenings and weekends are your time.
Relax, have fun, and enjoy yourself.

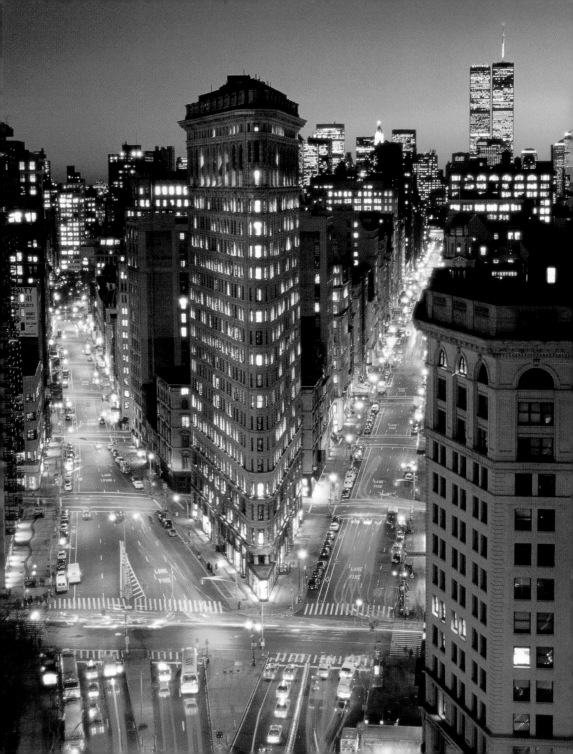

CHAPTER SEVEN

Leaving your work behind

The end of the working day is a strange in between time. It's all too easy simply to sling on your coat and race out of the office, keen to get on with the evening ahead. But pause a moment.

This is a threshold time of the day – psychologically, how you leave work is very important. It will have an effect not only on the evening in front of you but also on the next day at work. So spend five minutes recognizing and honouring this pivotal point of the day.

Five minutes planning and organizing yourself for the next working day will reap huge rewards in time and efficiency. Simple, easy techniques of time management help you to maximize your effectiveness, so you can leave work behind you with a clear conscience, knowing that all is in hand for tomorrow.

Your desk can be a shrine to personal creativity. Just a few minutes spent rearranging it and choosing your own power objects can transform it into an inspiring place to work.

Afterwards, it's worth spending a few minutes actively making the shift from work time to private time – switching, as it were, from your work persona to your private persona. If it's been a bad day, Reiki exercises will soothe and calm you, so you can let it all go and enjoy the evening ahead.

Easy yoga exercises and visualizations can help you cut the ties and make the break, while a simple "coming home" ritual makes your whole body and psyche aware that your working day is well and truly over.

Think ahead – plan for tomorrow

If you want to start the new day with energy, verve, and vigour, start planning the night before. This routine takes only five minutes at the end of each day but will save you hours the next. It also allows you to leave work feeling calm, centred, and in control.

FIVE MINUTE PLANNER
1 *Clear your desk. Check everything on your desk. Throw away all the trash. Copy important notes into a notebook or onto your computer. Put essential phone numbers in your address book. File away documents. Give your desk a polish with a duster that has a few drops of grapefruit aromatherapy oil on it.*

MAKE YOURSELF A DESK SHRINE
Take five minutes to transform your desk. A few well-chosen objects can turn your desk from a mere place of work to a shrine to creativity, inspiration, and enjoyable work. Choose objects that have meaning to you. The following are some suggestions:

★ *Crystals – they look attractive and augment your energy. Keep them on your computer or around your desk. Many have specific qualities: try citrine to give confidence, optimism, and to bring in money; rose quartz for harmony; bloodstone for decision-making; carnelian for motivation; tiger's eye for creativity; jade to help concentration and to keep things in perspective.*
★ *A candle or tea-light – this focuses the mind and keeps your concentration high.*
★ *Plants and flowers bring life and energy, provide good feng shui, and protect your environment (see pages 62–63).*

★ *Statues and figurines: a buddha for serenity; a goddess for groundedness; a dancing Shiva for energy; the Egyptian god Thoth for wisdom.*
★ *Beautiful pebbles, pieces of wood, shells, feathers – bring in the wonder of nature.*
★ *Photographs or framed postcards of people, places, or objects that inspire you. Frame motivational sayings or phrases too.*
★ *A bag of runestones, the I Ching or tarot cards for an instant office oracle.*
★ *Your own attractive mug or cup and saucer. Keep your water in a beautiful decanter and drink out of a special glass.*

2 *Check your diary. What do you need to do tomorrow? Make a list of all the appointments and tasks you need to complete. Are there any birthdays or important days coming up? What do you have planned for lunch?*

3 *Itemize your day. Use a desk diary divided into hours – or draw up your own plan for the day. First of all put down meetings and appointments. Remember to add in any travelling time. Now look at the tasks you need to do. How long will each take – realistically? Schedule in time for the most important – in descending order.*

4 *Plan "me" time. Try to schedule in a certain amount of time for yourself – whether it's for five minutes of yoga or relaxation (or any of the techniques in this book) – or to work on a long-term project.*

5 *Make a "spare time" list. List the things you would like to achieve – phone calls, writing letters, shopping, updating files. Keep this to one side.*

6 *Leave. You can now leave work knowing you have the next day well organized. Relax – it's all in hand.*

7 *The next day. Try to follow your schedule to the letter. If you find you have a spare 10 minutes before your next task, use it for your "spare time" list – or turn to one of the energy techniques in this book. Congratulations – you have made time!*

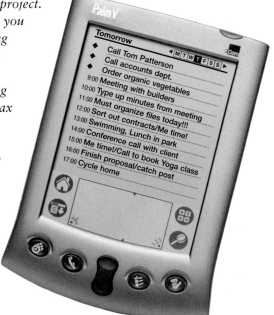

Cut the ties, make a break

Work's over – so why are you still thinking about it? If you find you are still mentally in the office when you're back at home, you need to cut the ties. Yoga stretching and breathing helps revitalize you, body and soul.

STRETCH AWAY THE DAY
Take off your shoes and stretch your toes. Take off your coat and anything restrictive, such as tight belts or jewelry. Find somewhere peaceful with enough space to stretch.

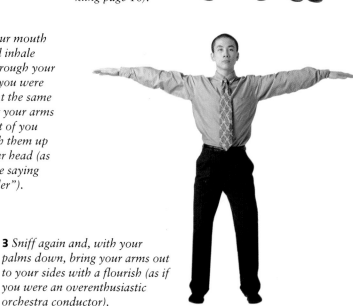

1 *Start by standing in the basic starting posture (see chi kung page 16).*

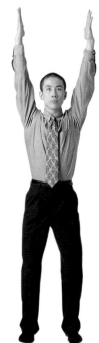

2 *Keep your mouth closed and inhale quickly through your nose as if you were sniffing. At the same time bring your arms up in front of you and stretch them up beside your head (as if you were saying "I surrender").*

3 *Sniff again and, with your palms down, bring your arms out to your sides with a flourish (as if you were an overenthusiastic orchestra conductor).*

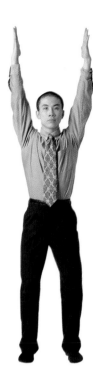

4 *Sniff a third time as your arms sweep back upwards.*

5 *Now at last you can exhale through your mouth with an explosive "Ha!" at the same time as you swing your arms downwards. Bend from the waist and knees so you hang down towards the floor like a floppy rag-doll. Relax your head, neck, shoulders, arms, and hands.*

Inhale through the nose as you swing your arms overhead and come back to a standing position, bringing your arms down to your sides.

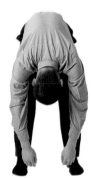

6 *Repeat steps 2 to 5 several times, letting the movements flow easily and smoothly. Let your gestures be as expansive as possible. Imagine you are throwing off all the cares of the day as you fling your arms out – up, to the sides, down to the floor. Let all the stress drop away. Let it go.*

Finally come back to the starting position and close your eyes. Check your energy. You should be feeling clear in your mind and invigorated in your body, ready for the evening ahead.

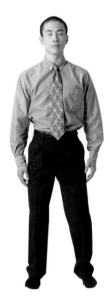

109

Shift your mood

Treat yourself with a short, simple ritual to help shift your mood when you get home: something that alerts your psyche that work is over, the evening is here.

COMING HOME RITUAL

1 Become aware, as you walk through your front door, that you are switching from the outer to the inner world. Hang up your coat, abandon your briefcase, take off your shoes – put on slippers or walk barefoot.
2 Take a refreshing shower. Put a couple of drops of lavender oil on a shower mitt (don't use in early pregnancy). Or try bergamot (but be careful if your skin is sensitive). As you shower, imagine washing away all the stresses of the day. You step out of the shower literally a different person.
3 Choose clothes that feel comfortable and fit your "home" persona. If you're staying in, choose something loose and casual. If you're going out, try an outfit that allows your true personality to show through. Express yourself.
4 Look at yourself in the mirror and tell yourself "I love myself, I approve of myself" over and over.

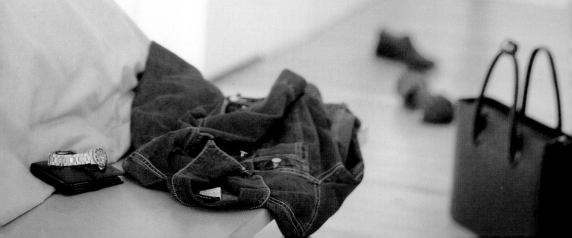

Banish a bad day

After a bad day soothe yourself with this breathing and touching exercise, which is based on Reiki, a Japanese form of spiritual healing. Use it to feel more centred, calm, and relaxed, or to throw off negative feelings.

REIKI RELAXATION

1 *Lie on your back, make yourself comfortable, and close your eyes. Start paying attention to your breath and follow its rhythm, noticing how it flows in and out.*

2 *Now put your hands on your body wherever you feel drawn to or where you feel tension. Use your intuition to locate the spot in your body that needs relaxation the most.*

3 *Now direct your breath to this place. Imagine you are breathing into that place. Visualize your breath as Universal Life Energy that is flowing through you. Imagine it collecting and expanding under your hands. Notice the feeling of relaxation and peace gradually spreading from the place beneath your hands throughout your entire body.*

4 *After about five minutes, place your hands on another part of your body and repeat step 3. You may find your breathing changes in this place. If so, just notice it and continue.*

5 *Move on to two further places in your body and charge them with energy.*

6 *Slowly open your eyes, stretch, and return to normal consciousness.*

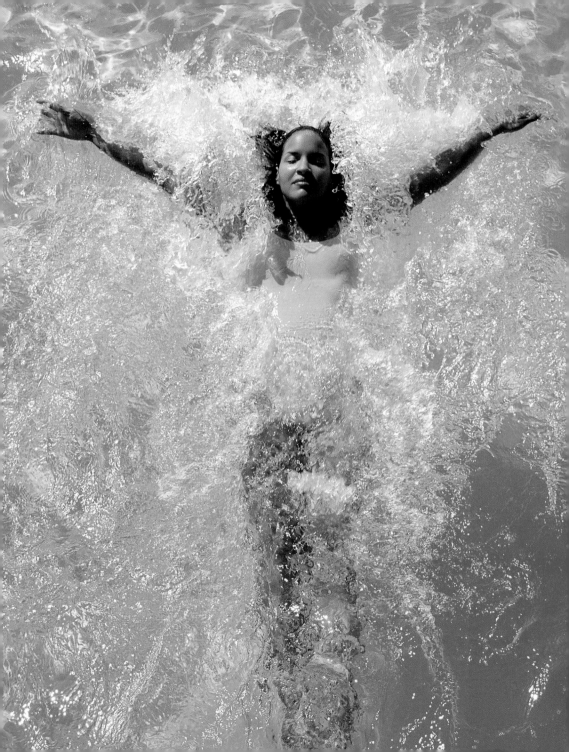

CHAPTER EIGHT

Time for yourself

You're home from work and the evening, or maybe even the weekend, stretches ahead. What will you do? How will you spend your free time? If you're going out, this chapter will help put you in the right frame of mind and body. If you're hoping for romance, there are even feng shui tips for creating the perfect setting for an intimate meal – guaranteed to put your partner in the mood.

If, on the other hand, you're staying in, resist the urge to slump in front of the TV all night – becoming a couch potato does nothing to raise your energy levels. Rather, take the opportunity to discover some hidden truths about your psyche; you could unleash your creativity and tackle your problems head-on. The benefits are enormous.

The process is great fun too. I'm not suggesting hours of turgid self-analysis but interesting ways of opening up your subconscious. Dancing can put you in touch with your innermost thoughts and feelings. If you've never painted, try art therapy – expressing yourself with paint can be both healing and revealing. You don't need to be artistic – in fact, the less

talented you are the more immediate your results will be!

You don't need to spend your whole evening or weekend engaged in these activities – unless you want to, of course. Some can offer remarkably speedy results. By the end of the evening, or before lunch on the weekend, you might have figured out your ideal exercise plan based on the principles of Ayurveda, or re-evaluated your diet according to the teachings of Tibetan medicine.

Use creative writing techniques to get in touch with your feelings and look back into your past, and you may start to write that bestselling novel or uncover the childhood cause of your weight problem. Not bad for a few hours' work.

Foods for moods

Are you in the mood for going out or staying in? The foods you eat can directly affect how you feel. So if you're going out you will need a high-energy meal to keep you going; if you're staying in you will want something to help you wind down.

THE CALM-DOWN, CHILL-OUT SUPPER

To help you calm down after a stressful day, choose foods that are high in carbohydrate, low in protein, and low in fat. A typical example would be:
■ White bean soup (see right).
■ Mixed green salad (calming).
■ Cornbread (reduces stress; induces relaxation).
If you're peckish before bedtime, choose a simple snack to induce relaxation and sleep – wholegrain cereal with low-fat or no-fat milk is ideal.

THE ENERGY BOOST

You're preparing for a night out on the town – you want to keep alert through the movie or give yourself enough energy to dance the night away. Choose a light, energy-packed meal or snack that is full of nutrients – high protein, low fat, balanced complex carbohydrate. For example:
■ Turkey breast salad, or warm chicken salad (see right) with mixed greens, grapes, and pine-nuts OR
■ Lentil dal with onions, tomatoes, and garlic – served with a small portion of wholegrain rice OR
■ Seafood stir-fry (avoid if you are pregnant).
■ Finish with fresh fruit, fruit salad (see right), or a fruit smoothie.

See Appendix (pages 152–153) for recipes.

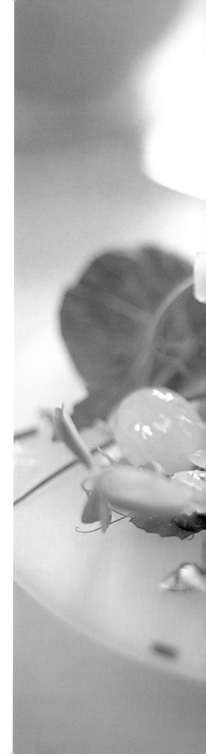

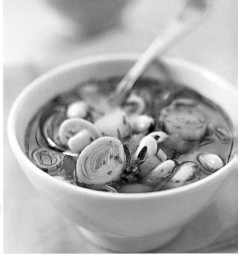

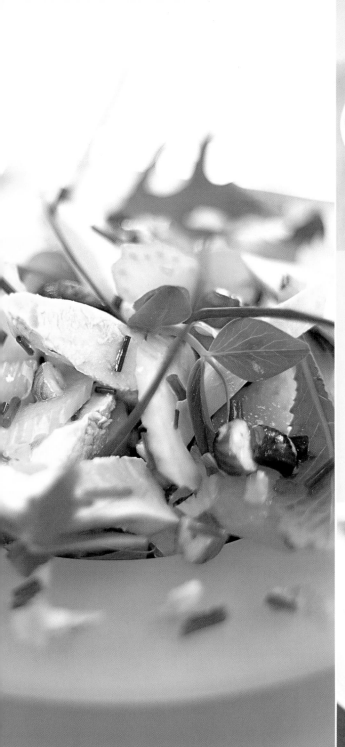

MOOD MEALS

The white bean soup (above) is a calm-down, chill-out dish. The beans and garlic help beat depression, while the pulses, onions, and potatoes relieve anxiety.

The warm chicken salad (left) is an energy-boosting meal, as is the fresh fruit salad (below).

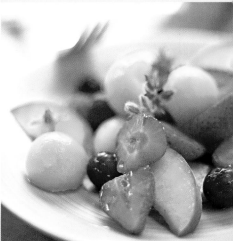

Prepare to party

Dancing liberates both body and soul. A good dance can directly engage your emotions and put you in touch with your deepest feelings, your most hidden thoughts. Biodanza is a dance therapy in which every exercise and its accompanying music is carefully planned to have a precise physiological effect. This home Biodanza class provides you with a tingle of energy and puts you in the perfect mood to party.

HOME DANCE CLASS

1 *Walk around the room feeling connected with your body. Feel your feet connecting firmly with the ground; let your arms swing naturally and keep your head up high. Gradually let your movement become more fluid, more vital, more exuberant.*
2 *Put on music with a strong but fluid melody. Dance in any way you choose but remain aware of your chest and heart area and dance "into" that area.*
3 *Change the music for something with a firm rhythm and let your pelvic region govern your movements.*
4 *Keep the rhythmic music on and play with finding your "own" dance. Forget notions of what dancing should look like; don't worry about proper steps or movements. Allow the music to dance you: jump in the air or roll on the floor – it doesn't matter!*
5 *Now try "giving" your dance to someone else. One of you should sit on the floor and "receive" the dance while you dance for her/him. If you are alone, imagine you are dancing for someone special and pretend they are sitting in front of you. Maintain eye contact all the way through the exercise. Then swap over and "receive" their dance.*

Once you've found your "own" dance, try "giving" it to someone else. It's fun and very rewarding.

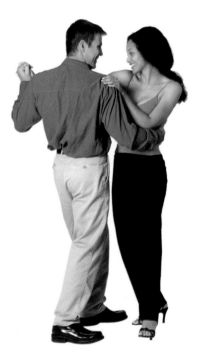

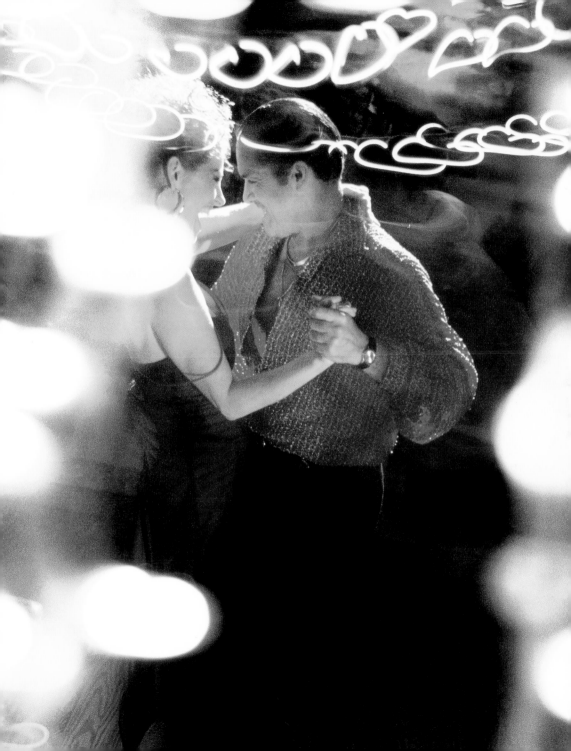

Resolve your problems

Painting and drawing might seem like child's play but picking up a brush or a pencil could be the best thing you've done in your adult life. You don't need to be Picasso: art therapists insist that the simple act of putting marks on the paper can be a healing – and revealing – process.

FREEFORM ART THERAPY

1 Look at your paints (or felt pens, crayons, etc.). To which colours are you drawn? Don't rationalize, just follow your instinct. Pour them onto your palette.
2 Pick up a paintbrush or scraper and start to paint. You may know exactly what you want to paint or you may just make marks on the paper. Don't criticize yourself – just do what seems right.
3 Keep painting and see which images emerge. Sometimes quite unexpected forms appear in the work. What do they remind you of?
4 You may want to sit down and just look at your painting. What is it saying to you? Does it show more about how you think or how you feel about your life? What are the themes and questions in it? Even if the answer is "a big mess" maybe that has a resonance in your life.
5 How do you feel in your body after painting? Pay attention to any aches and pains or feelings.
6 Try dialoguing with your painting. "Talk" or write to the images in it. What do they reply?
7 Do you feel you now need to do another painting? If so, go ahead. If not, date your painting and keep it – look at it in a week or so and see if any further ideas come to mind.

> **GETTING STARTED**
> *If you find it hard to get started, you may like to try these suggestions:*
> ★ *Paint with your nondominant hand – this bypasses the conscious mind entirely.*
> ★ *Try painting to music. Put on a piece that moves you and see what happens.*
> ★ *Try painting blindfolded! You may be surprised at the results.*

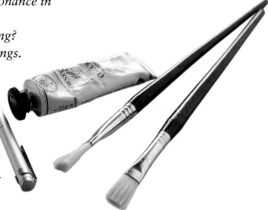

Unleash your creativity

Writing can act as a potent form of self-therapy, illuminating the past and helping us understand ourselves in the present. Writing freely can release emotional blocks, free creativity, and help us in almost every area of our lives.

GETTING IN TOUCH WITH YOUR FEELINGS

1 Take one of the following opening lines and complete the sentence. "I want…" or "I don't want…" or "I wish I could…" or "In an ideal world…."
2 Then write the same opening line and complete it in a different way. Continue like this for five minutes. Don't think or judge – just write whatever comes into your head. The repetition helps to release feelings – you may find some surprises.

TAPPING THE SUBCONSCIOUS

Free association – putting down the first words that come into your head and then following wherever they lead – will allow your deepest feelings to surface. Don't be tempted to think about what you're writing. It doesn't matter if what you write seems trivial or silly. If personal, private, uncertain, or difficult feelings come up, give yourself permission to write them down. You don't have to show this to anyone.

There are various ways of starting off. You might start writing for five minutes, with one of these:
"I'll never forget…"
"All I really wanted in my life was to…"
"The thing I hated most was…"
"If I'm really honest…"

BACK INTO MEMORY
This exercise allows old childhood feelings, possibly hurtful, to emerge safely.
★ *Write about something from your past – a beloved toy, a favourite pet, a house, or place you remember well.*
★ *Use an old photograph as a trigger for writing about your past. Think back to how life was then. Who were your friends? Where did you live? How did you feel?*
★ *Write a profile of someone from your past – a deceased parent perhaps? A childhood friend? An old teacher…*

Discover your ideal exercise

Find a form of exercise you actively enjoy and you are onto a winner. Exercise not only tones the body, it also helps your mind. The key to successful exercise is to find something you really love. Ayurveda, the ancient Indian mind-body medicine, can help because it divides us all into three basic constitutional types. Turn to the table on the right and find out which Ayurvedic type you are.

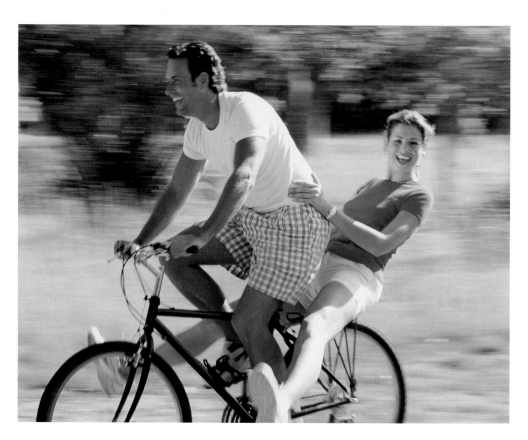

AYURVEDA AND EXERCISE
The table below will help you identify which of the three Ayurvedic types you are – vata (air), pitta (fire), or kapha (earth). The sports in the "natural inclinations" column are those that come most naturally to you. To balance your nature, try one of the exercises from the "sports to balance" column.

TYPE	VATA	PITTA	KAPHA
DESCRIPTION	Small-framed with an active mind and restless body. You talk a lot, ask a lot of questions, and can't seem to sit still. Quick, light, and agile, you are not very muscular and don't have a lot of endurance.	Fiery, aggressive, competitive, and vocal, you often tend to assume the leadership role. You are usually strong, medium-framed, and well coordinated.	Kapha types usually have heavier frames than Vata or Pitta, with strong bodies and high endurance. You are slower moving, slower speaking, and easygoing by nature.
NATURAL INCLINATIONS	Running, sprinting, any kind of track sports (e.g. hurdles, long jump, high jump, relay).	The more competitive the sport the better (e.g. tennis, squash).	Sports requiring endurance and power. You do well with team sports and thrive under the motivation of others.
SPORTS TO BALANCE	Anything that will soothe and calm your restless nature. Low-impact jogging or aerobics, walking, hiking, cycling, and swimming.	Anything that isn't so intensely competitive. Cycling, swimming, skiing, or golf but also yoga, tai chi, and chi kung.	You need speeding up, enlivening, so any fast sports that require endurance, such as tennis, rowing, running, or high-intensity aerobics are all excellent for kapha.

Balance your diet with Tibetan medicine

Tibetan medicine specifies three "humours" – air, bile, and phlegm – and each of us has a predisposition to one of them (see table opposite). Air controls breathing, speech, and muscular activity, as well as the nervous system, thought processes, and your emotional attitude. Bile governs heat in the body, the liver, and the digestive tract, while phlegm controls the amount of mucus in the body and regulates the immune system.

When diagnosing an imbalance of the humours, a Tibetan doctor will study your pulse. An experienced physician can identify up to 95 percent of all known diseases from the pulse alone, indeed some can anticipate the life expectancy of an individual from their pulse alone. A Tibetan doctor will usually request a urine sample to confirm a diagnosis and analyze its colour, odour, sedimentation, and persistence of bubbles. The shape, colour, and coating of your tongue are also significant.

A Tibetan doctor will then ask you many questions concerning your general lifestyle, behaviour, and diet and will normally recommend modifications to all three depending upon your imbalance of humours. Diet is of particular importance as all foods affect the humours in different ways and can either cause or exacerbate the domination of air, bile, or phlegm. A Tibetan physician will also advise you how much you should eat, when, and how often.

Use the table (opposite) to find out which foods are most suited to you. Try following the dietary advice for your predominant humour to keep yourself fit and well – and increase your energy and wellbeing.

WHAT'S YOUR TIBETAN TYPE?

Identify which type you are by comparing the symptoms you have a tendency towards with one of the humours below. Collect urine in a clear jar first thing in the morning. Check its appearance to confirm which type you are (urine analysis is a classic Tibetan diagnostic tool). Then follow the dietary regime to balance you.

HUMOUR	AIR	BILE	PHLEGM
SYMPTOMS	Stress, insomnia, constipation, back pains, dry skin. Dizziness, shivering, sighing, pain in hips and shoulder blades, humming in ears. Restless mind.	Easily hot and sweaty. Thirsty, bitter taste in the mouth, pains in the upper body. Feverish; diarrhea or vomiting. Wake up feeling bright and cheerful but by midday are feeling irritable.	Lethargic, frequent indigestion or belching; distended stomach; cold feet. Find it hard to lose weight. Prone to oversleeping; fond of the odd nap.
URINE	Watery, almost transparent	Yellow or brownish	Very pale and foaming
DIET TO BALANCE	Avoid cold foods such as salads and ice cream or make sure you have a hot drink beforehand (e.g. ginger tea). Base your diet around chicken, meat broths, cheese, onions, carrots, garlic and spices, spinach and greens.	Cool light foods such as salads and yogurt, and plenty of cool water. Avoid hot, spicy foods, nuts, alcohol, and red meat.	Warm the digestion with ginger (not in early pregnancy), cardamom, nutmeg (use sparingly). Also peppermint (avoid if breastfeeding). Don't eat too much sugar-rich fruit if you're trying to lose weight. Avoid dairy products.

Conjure up romance

It takes more than just fine food and the odd candle for a romantic dinner for two. What you need is the subtle power of feng shui.

AN INTIMATE DINNER TABLE

1 *Choose a round, wooden table – not too large – it needs to feel intimate.*

2 *Cover it with a purple, lilac, or mauve table cloth in an unusual fabric, such as velvet or silk.*

3 *Seat yourself at right angles to your partner so you can talk easily.*

4 *Candlelight is essential. Choose a candlestick no more than three inches (8 cm) high so it does not create a barrier. Set it on a small, polished display mirror.*

5 *Place a vase of flowers on the other side of the table so it doesn't come between you. Choose a purple or lilac-coloured vase and soft, romantic, scented flowers. Avoid harsh, sculptural flowers or any with spiky leaves or petals.*

6 *A champagne bucket (with champagne!) also helps the mood. Crystal flutes catch the candlelight and spread beneficial energy.*

7 *Incorporate on the table all the five elements traditional to Chinese philosophy – a decanter of wine or water (water); cutlery (metal); candles or an overhead light (fire); the table (wood); and the glasses (earth). Including every element promotes balance.*

8 *Light music in the background is fine but make sure it is suitable and does not interfere with conversation. Light classical or jazz is usually a good choice.*

9 *Keep lighting soft and balanced – you need to see what you're eating but not in a harsh, clinical light.*

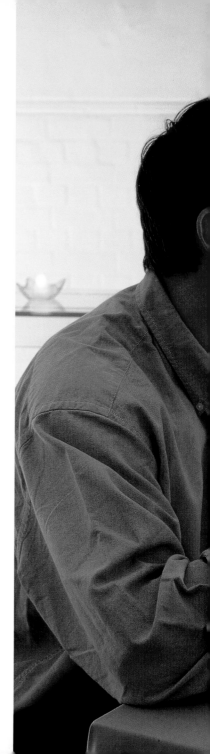

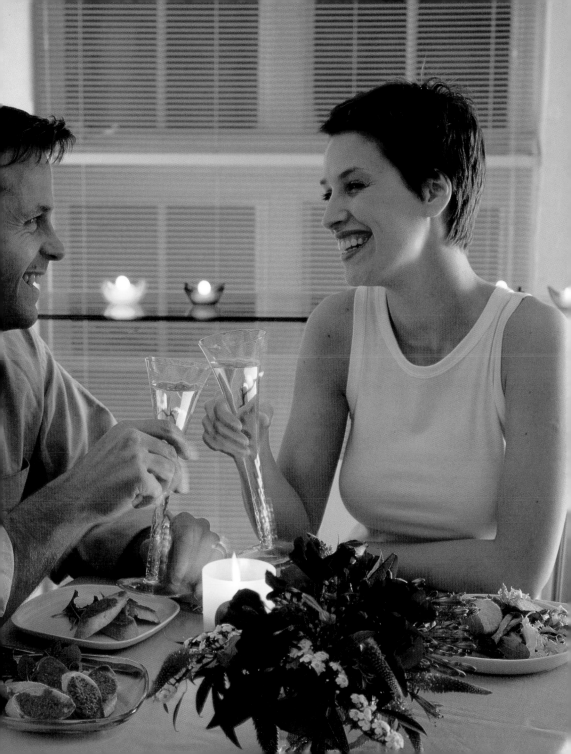

Go within and find peace

There is nothing like yoga to help you relax at the end of the day. Yoga stretches out mind and body, soothing the psyche and balancing your energy. Taking five minutes to wind down with this lovely sequence will set you up for the evening – whatever you choose to do afterwards.

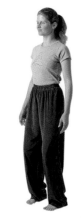

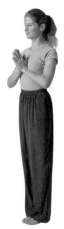

10 *Now work back through all these steps from 8 to 1, ending by placing your palms together in front of your chest in the sign of salutation.*

1 *Stand in the basic starting posture (see chi kung page 16).*

9 *Inhale gently and stretch out on the floor, face down. Then straighten your arms, pushing your upper body backwards.*

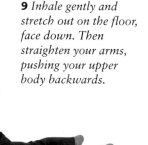

8 *Exhale gently and bring your arms and torso down and forwards, lowering your buttocks to rest on your calves. Bend forwards, touching your head on the floor.*

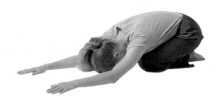

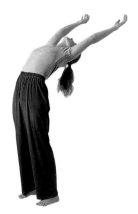

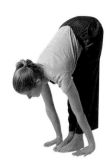

3 *Exhale gently, slowly bringing the arms forwards. Bend your torso forwards, keeping your legs straight, and touch the floor with your palms.*

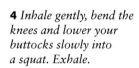

2 *Inhale gently and raise both arms up over the head, gently bending the upper body and head backwards as far as comfortable.*

4 *Inhale gently, bend the knees and lower your buttocks slowly into a squat. Exhale.*

7 *Inhale gently and bring your right knee back to rest on the floor beside your left knee. Kneeling, raise your arms up over your head and gently bend your body back as far as is comfortable.*

5 *Inhale gently. Extend the left leg back with the knee touching the floor. Raise your arms over your head and bend your upper body.*

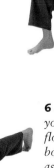

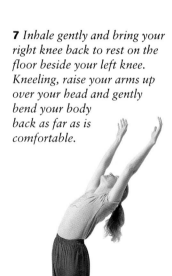

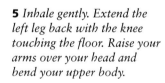

6 *Exhale gently, bringing your palms down to the floor, and stretch your body forwards as far as possible.*

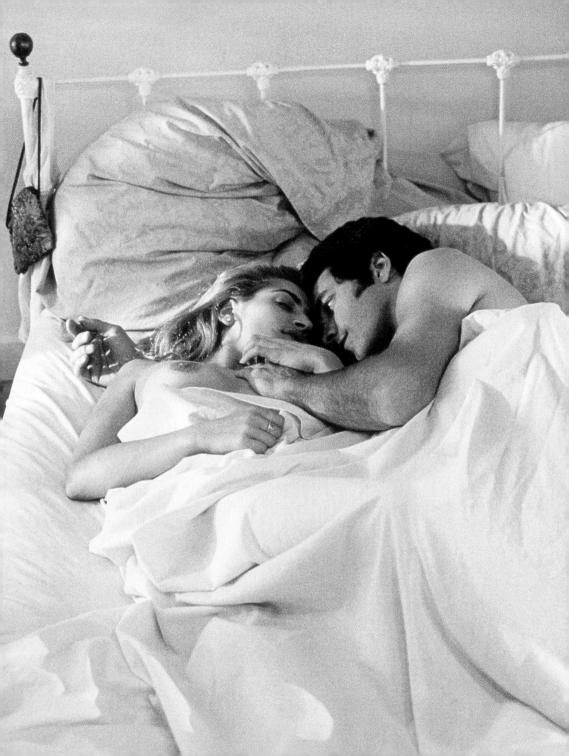

CHAPTER NINE

End of the day

The day is drawing to a close. This is the time when you want to bring your energy down slowly and gently as you approach the borders of sleep. It's a time of reflection, of summation, of soft gentle energy. Turn bedtime into a ritual – make it special.

First of all spend some time transforming your bedroom into a haven of peace and quiet, an embracing sanctuary. It should be the familiar place where you can retreat and relax from the stresses and strains of the day: a bolt-hole, a place of restoration, sensuality, and dreams.

Indulge in this slowing towards slumber time. Don't just brush your teeth and jump into bed: give yourself the luxury of a long bath, using one of the special recipes to promote sweet dreams – or banish a cold.

Feeling sluggish and need a detox? Use the healing energies of water and the power of hydrotherapy to rid your body of the toxins it has accumulated during the day.

Lie back and enjoy a sensuous full-body massage with your partner or, together, use reflexology techniques in a foot massage that will calm and relax you.

And does your face still show the cares of the day? Then treat yourself to a rejuvenating facial massage – a natural facelift. If you're in the mood for intimacy and romance, learn how to make sex really shimmer with an exciting and ancient Tantric ritual.

If your energy is still running high after a hectic day, there are suggestions for preparing for sleep and for soothing insomnia. If you're feeling tense and stressed five-minute tension-busters will soon transform you, mind and body. Finally, as you drift into sleep, learn how to promote dreaming and to use your dreams to bring you peace and understanding.

Sleep tight. Sweet dreams.

Sleep soundly – the bedroom sanctuary

Transform your bedroom into a refuge of calm and tranquillity and you will find you sleep more deeply, which, in turn, will allow you to awake refreshed and full of energy. By following simple rules from feng shui, the ancient Chinese art of placement, you will be able to relax after a tough day's work.

FENG SHUI FOR BETTER BEDROOMS

■ Clear out all the clutter from your bedroom – and keep it out. Psychologists point out that if your environment is cluttered, your mind will be unable to relax. You will subconsciously be worried about the mess and what needs doing.

■ Try to avoid working in your bedroom. If this is impossible, place your desk or workspace behind a screen, so you cannot be reminded of work while you are in bed.

■ Turn out wardrobes and cupboards regularly – donate unworn or unwanted clothes to charity shops or dress agencies.

■ Place your bed so you can see the door – ideally diagonally opposite the door. Do not have your headboard backing onto a window or doorway.

■ Keep furniture, such as tables and chairs, soft and rounded – avoid sharp edges or points.

■ Avoid big mirrors. Keep mirrors small and preferably round or oval. Do not have a mirror opposite your bed – it may cause insomnia or bad dreams.

■ Choose colours wisely – include pinks and reds for romance, soft blues for relaxation. Cushions and candles can be bright pinks and reds, but always avoid dark, heavy colours.

BOOKS & ORNAMENTS
Keep bookshelves out of the bedroom – they distract the mind with the weight of all those books! And keep any ornaments restrained as well – a few well-chosen ones are far better than a whole collection that makes the bedroom busy and gathers dust.

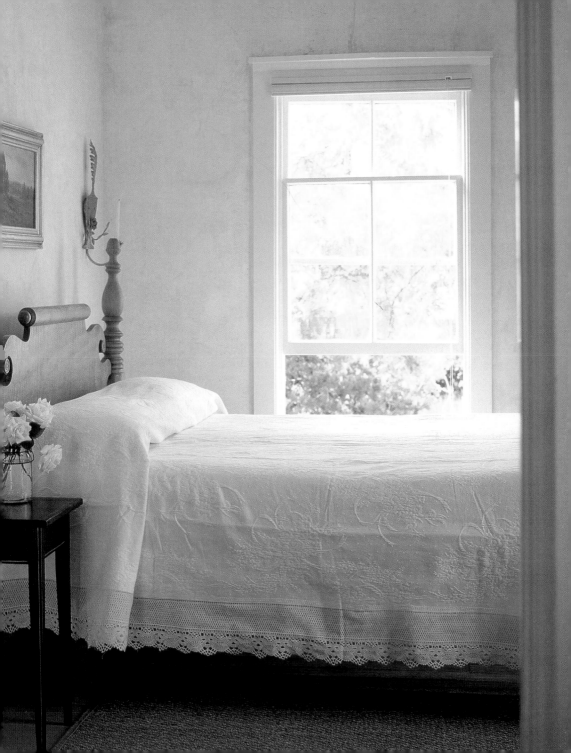

Your pleasure zone

Remember that your bedroom should be a place of rest and relaxation.

■ Pile the bed with sumptuous cushions and pillows (stuff them with herbs such as lavender and geranium for a good night's sleep).
■ Choose soft, gentle lighting. Avoid harsh overhead lights and pick soft bedside lamps or uplifters instead. Candles are ideal, especially those made with pure aromatherapy oils (rather than synthetic fragrances) to add delicious scents: lavender or chamomile are wonderful for relaxation and promoting sleep. Ylang ylang and sandalwood will make the bedroom enticing for romance. But put out the candles before you sleep.
■ Fresh flowers make your bedroom special. Plant window boxes with night-scented stocks, lavender, and chamomile for sweet dreams throughout the summer. Fill vases with sweet-scented, old-fashioned roses, hyacinths, lilies, or sweet peas. Make posies of herbs that not only smell sweet but also deter insects.
■ Buy an aromatherapy burner and scent your bedroom with your favourite scents – try ylang ylang, sandalwood, lavender, geranium for starters. Pop a few drops of lavender oil on a tissue and tuck it by your pillow. Remember, don't overdo the ylang ylang – it can cause headaches and nausea; and don't use lavender in the early months of pregnancy.
■ Balance light and shade. In the morning, it's lovely to maximize the light but at night you need darkness for a good sleep. If you have curtains, consider shifting the mood as the seasons change – comforting, warm velvets or plaids for winter and cool, crisp linen or floaty voile for summer.

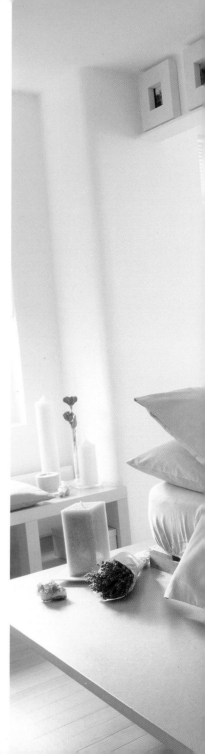

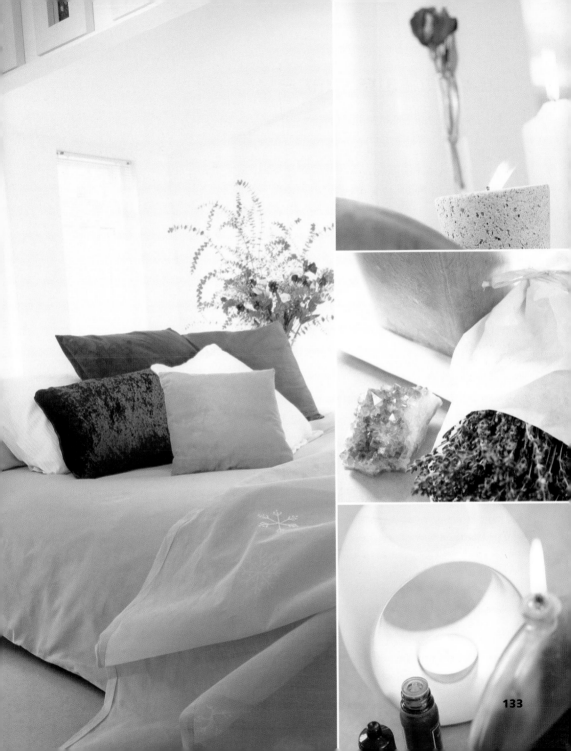

Create a safe space

Your bedroom should be a sanctuary from the world: a safe, secure place in which you leave the cares of the day behind. However, health problems can result from unseen dangers in our bedrooms – from allergies to headaches, from memory loss to depression.

SAFETY-PROOF YOUR BED
Chemicals used to treat fabric and materials in beds and bedlinen can give off fumes and may cause allergies, insomnia, tiredness, coughing, skin rashes, headaches, and throat and eye irritation.
■ Choose iron or untreated solid wood bedframes. Antique bedframes are an alternative, since most formaldehyde gas will have evaporated after 10 years. However, there is evidence that iron bedframes may exacerbate electric fields in the room.
■ Choose sheets made from unbleached percale or "organic" cotton for summer. Cotton flannel sheets are ideal for winter. If you can afford it, check out natural linen sheets.
■ Think about switching to a pure cotton mattress – without flame-resistant finishes. Futon mattresses are also safe. Choose cotton-filled pillows.
■ If you're sensitive to dust mites, buy anti-allergy mattress and pillow covers.

BANISH EMFS
EMFs (electromagnetic fields) are produced by electricity and emitted by any appliance that is powered by electricity. EMFs have been linked with a range of health problems, from headaches and nausea to brain tumours and breast cancer.
■ If possible, keep all electric appliances out of the

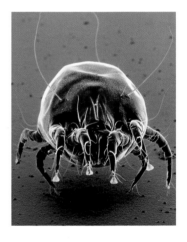

Dust mites carried in dust can cause allergies such as asthma in sensitive people. A particular problem in standard mattresses and pillow cases, the effect of dust mites can be minimized by specially designed covers.

bedroom, particularly TVs and computers. If this isn't possible, make sure they are as far away as possible from your bed – EMFs are much weaker more than 3 feet (1 metre) away.

■ Don't fall asleep with the TV on – switch it off and unplug it.

■ Swap your electric alarm clock for a battery-powered or old-fashioned wind-up version.

■ Electric blankets can expose you to EMFs at night. Make sure you unplug yours before going to sleep or, even better, warm your bed with hot water bottles.

WATCH OUT FOR GEOPATHIC STRESS

Streams deep underground, large deposits of minerals, or geological faults in the substrata of the planet create abnormal energy fields. These fields create "bad spots" in our homes and workplaces where they are stressful to us by interfering with our own energy.

There is increasing evidence that the resulting geopathic stress (GS) may contribute to many disturbances in our lives, including divorce, nightmares, and cancer. Sufferers from GS feel tired constantly and get irritable easily. Ailments, aches, and pains never seem to go away. If you think you may be a sufferer:

■ Place cork tiles under your bed for a few weeks. If you start to feel better, try moving your bed.

■ Switch on a hairdryer and run it all over you with the side of the dryer touching your body. It may help to reduce the effects of GS although you shouldn't consider it as a preventative. Try it once a week.

A hairdryer, an unlikely tool for reducing the effects of GS.

Massage with a partner

Massage is simply the superlative way to relax and let go of the day, to focus your senses and become deeply aware of your body's responses. Go by your instincts, and ask your partner if he or she is enjoying it.

RELAXING TOGETHER

1 *Light candles and put on relaxing music. Burn some relaxing essential oils (lavender or chamomile) or romantic oils (sandalwood or ylang ylang) in a burner. Caution: avoid lavender in early pregnancy and chamomile in the first four months of pregnancy. Too much ylang ylang can cause headaches and nausea.*
2 *Use eight drops of your essential oil in 4 teaspoons (15–20ml) of a base oil (sweet almond or soya oil).*
3 *Massage in a slow, steady rhythm with the right amount of pressure for your partner.*
4 *Start on the back, with your thumbs on either side of the spine, fingers pointing towards the neck. Let your hands glide slowly up the body and around the shoulders. Draw your hands lightly down the side of the back to your starting position.*
5 *Move on to the shoulders, arms, and legs. Gently knead fleshy areas, such as hips and thighs: lift, squeeze, and roll the skin between the thumb and fingers of one hand and glide it towards the other.*
6 *Curl your fingers into loose fists. With the fingers (not the knuckles), work all over the body.*
7 *Make small circles with your thumbs on shoulders, palms of the hands, soles of the feet, and chest.*
8 *Cup your hands, and with quick, light movements move over the skin as if you were beating a drum.*
9 *End your massage with slow, smooth, stroking movements.*

> **CAUTIONS**
> *Don't massage anyone with:*
> ★ *a contagious disease, fever, or a high temperature*
> ★ *a skin infection, serious bruising, or inflammation*
> ★ *a bad back pain*
> ★ *phlebitis or thrombosis*
> ★ *diabetes, epilepsy, high or low blood pressure, or any heart problems*
> ★ *varicose veins – although the rest of the body can be massaged*
> ★ *a woman in the first four months of pregnancy*

Enhance the effects of your massage with some relaxing essential oils.

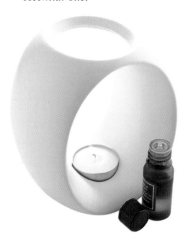

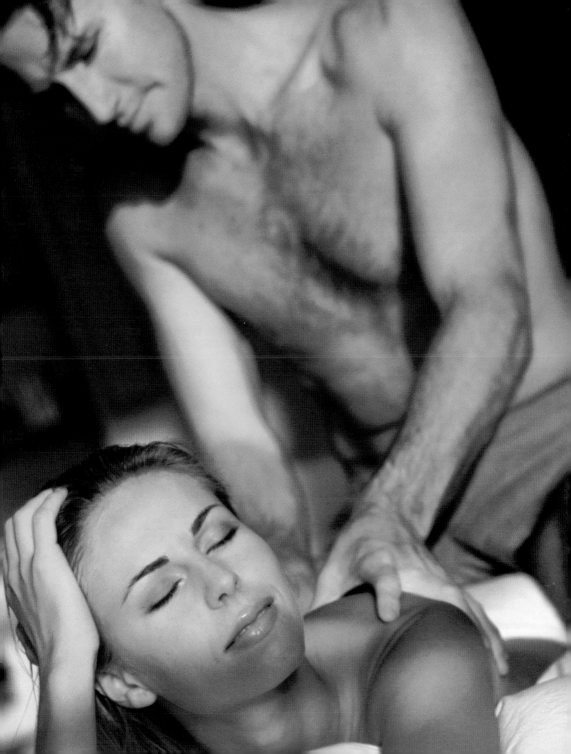

Be soothed!

There is nothing quite as relaxing as a gentle foot massage. When you combine it with the power of reflexology, you have a recipe for the perfect wind-down routine. Ask your partner to perform this sequence on you – or adapt it for use on yourself. It uses sesame oil which, according to Ayurvedic teaching, is very soothing at night. If you're allergic to sesame, then try coconut oil.

> **CAUTION**
> ★ *Only use lightest foot massage on a pregnant woman – and omit step 6*
> ★ *Only a highly qualified reflexologist should perform reflexology during pregnancy.*

RELAXING FOOT MASSAGE

1 *Gently warm some plain, not roasted, sesame oil in a bowl by standing it in another bowl of hot water. Massage the right foot first. Pour some oil into the palm of your hand and then gently massage it into the foot. Use large movements to spread the oil well.*

2 *Now cover the foot in more detail, making small circling movements with the pad of your thumb. Work over the sole (firmly if the person is ticklish), the heels, and the ankles.*

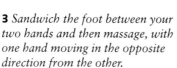

3 *Sandwich the foot between your two hands and then massage, with one hand moving in the opposite direction from the other.*

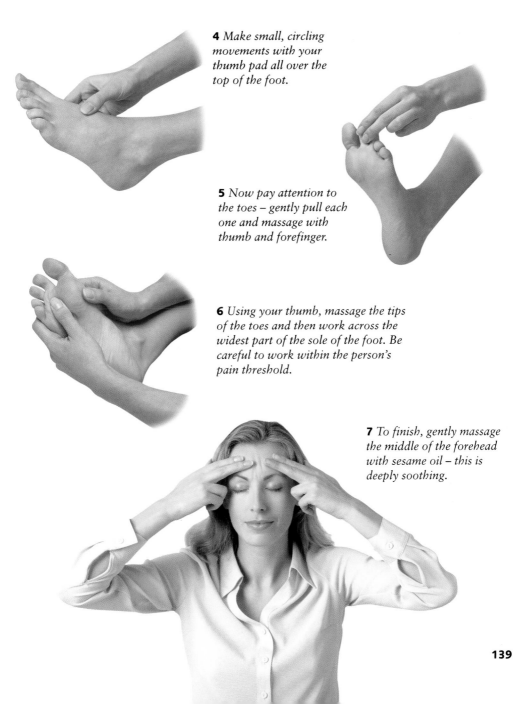

4 *Make small, circling movements with your thumb pad all over the top of the foot.*

5 *Now pay attention to the toes – gently pull each one and massage with thumb and forefinger.*

6 *Using your thumb, massage the tips of the toes and then work across the widest part of the sole of the foot. Be careful to work within the person's pain threshold.*

7 *To finish, gently massage the middle of the forehead with sesame oil – this is deeply soothing.*

Sound sleep

If you are feeling slightly run-down, or think you might be getting a cold, try the Epsom salts bath. It is also deeply and profoundly relaxing – use it just before going to bed. The herbal and aromatherapy bath below is a perfect way to unwind after a tough day, promising good sleep and sweet dreams.

> **CAUTION**
> *Avoid Epsom salts baths if you have heart trouble, if you are diabetic, or are feeling tired or weak.*

EPSOM SALTS BATH

1 *Run a warm bath and dissolve about 16 oz (450 g) of Epsom salts in the water. Get in and relax for as long as you are comfortable while you drink a cup of hot peppermint tea, which increases perspiration and replaces lost fluids. If you're breastfeeding drink thyme instead.*

2 *Be careful as you get out – you may feel light-headed. Do not rub yourself dry. Wrap up in several large towels and go to bed. Don't forget to wrap your feet up warmly.*

3 *When you wake up, unwrap the towels and give yourself a good sponge-down with warm water. Then rub yourself really vigorously until you're dry.*

SWEET DREAMS

1 *Take the following dried herbs – 3 tablespoons each of chamomile, linden blossom, cowslip, vervain, and woodruff and boil for twenty minutes in about 5 pints (3 litres) of water.*

2 *Meanwhile prepare your bathroom. Light candles around your bath. Put on some soft, relaxing music (use a battery-powered machine – not one plugged into the mains). Burn lavender oil in a diffuser.*

3 *Your bath should be pleasantly warm – not too hot or too cool. Strain the herbs through a piece of muslin* *and add the decoction to your bath. Add 4 drops of lavender or chamomile essential oil.*

4 Climb into your bath. Place a towel behind your head. Now gently close your eyes and imagine you are lying in a magical pool – perhaps deep in the woods or on a gorgeous beach or in a beautiful temple.

5 Visualize the water drawing out all the stresses and strains of your day, banishing all the negativity and doubts you have. They simply vaporize and disappear.

6 Lie and enjoy the feeling of total relaxation. If you like, you can tie up the muslin into a bag and use it as a herbal flannel.

DETOX YOUR SYSTEM

Water is a wonderful healer – and a powerful way of detoxing your body, especially when it's hot. Whenever you are feeling run-down or sluggish, try this body-pack technique to sweat away the toxic debris from your body.

Detox body pack

Body packs (they're also called body wraps) will make you sweat – just like a sauna or steam bath – and help you get rid of toxins from your body.

1 Completely cover a cotton sheet in cold water. Then squeeze out as much water as you can so the sheet is cold on the skin but doesn't drip.

2 Cover your bed (or a couch) with a large piece of plastic. Then spread your damp sheet on top of the plastic.

3 Take off all your clothes and lie down on the sheet. Ask one of your friends or your partner to prepare three hot water bottles and to put one by your chest, one beside your waist, and one next to your feet. Then ask them to wrap the sheet around you, leaving only your head exposed.

4 This may seem daunting but relax and steam yourself for three whole hours. After 10 to 15 minutes you'll probably sweat a great deal and then don't be surprised if you fall asleep. Despite all the moisture the sheet will be nearly dry when the treatment is complete – and will probably be discoloured by the toxins.

Look younger

This massage stimulates and tones the tiny muscles of your face, acting like a natural face-lift. Treat yourself every night and notice the difference.

REJUVENATING MASSAGE

1 *Put five to ten drops of oil in the palm of your hands and apply it all over the face. Choose almond oil (fine for all skins), olive oil (ideal for very dry skin), or jojoba oil (good for sensitive and oily skins).*

2 *Put a small amount of facial exfoliator (two heaped teaspoons of fine oatmeal with two teaspoons of double cream) in the palm of your hand and apply it to the face, neck, and ears, with a light action using the pads of your fingers. Rinse with warm water.*

3 *Using the balls of your fingers, polish the skin with a circular, gliding motion. Begin with the neck, then move along the jaw, cheeks, ears, backs of ears, around the nose, forehead, and temples. Rinse with warm water.*

4 *Use your middle finger (unless otherwise directed) and work clockwise for 30 seconds on each of these points: the middle of the chin, both corners of the mouth to the mid-point between your nose, and the cupid's bow of your upper lip.*

5 *At the centre of your cheekbones push upwards and massage. Press gently on the eye orbit bone above your cheekbones – use your forefinger and do not massage.*

6 *With your thumbs press upwards on the inner edge of your eyebrows. Pinch along each eyebrow from the inside to the outside edge.*

7 *Massage the temples gently.*

8 *Apply a small amount of aloe vera gel all over the face. Finish with your own special moisturizer.*

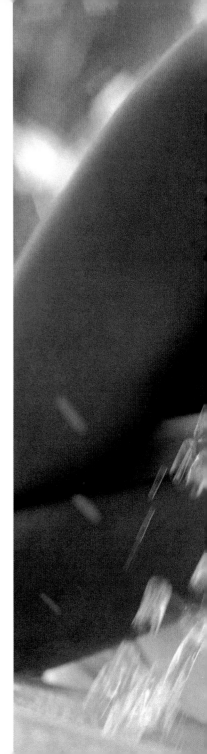

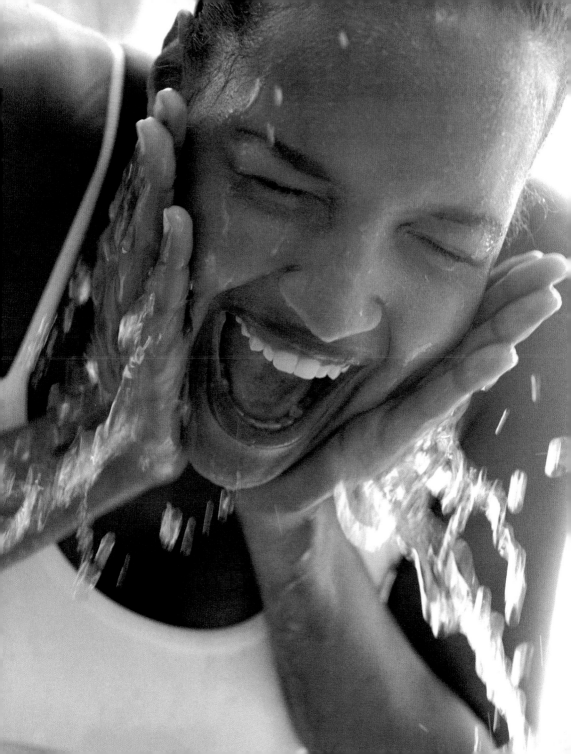

Banish bugs and flu

At the first signs of colds or flu, jump straight into this healing bath. It should help to stop a cold in its tracks.

COLD-BEATING BATH

1 *Make up your oil: add two drops each of lavender, bergamot, and tea-tree essential oils to four teaspoons of carrier oil (ie sweet almond, jojoba, or avocado oil) or full fat milk. Add the mixture to a hot bath and disperse the oil. Caution: avoid lavender in early pregnancy and bergamot if your skin is sensitive.*
2 *Get in and relax for at least 20 minutes.*

> **NOTE**
> *Some people find essential oils irritate the skin – sample the oil you've made up on your wrist before jumping into a whole bath containing it.*

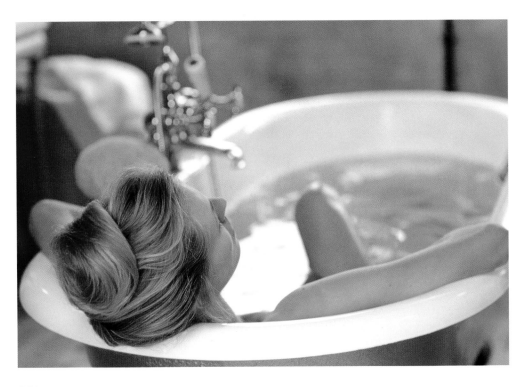

Arouse your sensuality

Need some help to get in the mood before a night of passion? Ignite your ardour with these aphrodisiac fixes based on working the pressure points in shiatsu.

PASSSION RAISER

1 *Start with a general back massage (see pages 136-137). If you like, use a sensual massage blend – mix four drops of ylang ylang or sandalwood oil in a teaspoon of peach kernel or sweet almond oil.*
2 *Now focus on the acupressure points at the base of the spine. With your thumbs, work gently but firmly up the spine from the top of the buttocks to a point parallel with the top of the hip. Don't press too hard on the spine. Press firmly and hold for about seven seconds, release and wait five seconds, then repeat.*
3 *Now turn your partner over. If you are working on a man, massage firmly with fingers and thumbs around the upper thighs into the groin and pelvic bone. This area is rich in pressure points so you can't go far wrong! If working on a woman, use pressure on the point that lies directly on top of the pubic bone (allies with the G-spot inside the vagina). Then turn your attention to the series of points that run either side of the breast bone (the heart points).*

To arouse the sensuality of a man, you need to focus on the pressure points around the upper thighs.

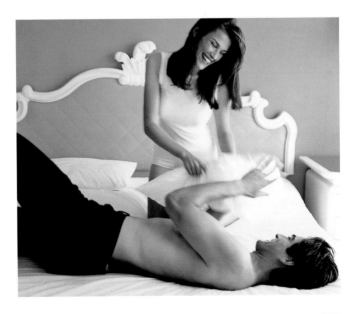

Enjoy super sex

The ancient Indian art of Tantra teaches union with God through lovemaking. It involves visualization, breathing, meditation, and practical sex. This ritual, based on the Tantric ceremony known as *maithuna*, can give surprisingly intense results very swiftly.

TANTRIC MAITHUNA

1 *Prepare your bedroom with care: fresh sheets and exotic silk or satin coverings over the bed; soft music, fresh flowers; burn aphrodisiac essential oils, such as ylang ylang and sandalwood; light red candles.*
2 *Prepare a tray with small, exotic nibbles (nothing too heavy) and wine (but don't overdo the alcohol).*
3 *Bath and dress in light, flowing clothes.*
4 *Spend time simply enjoying each other's company, talking, eating, and drinking together. Touch and caress each other, gazing deep into each other's eyes.*
5 *To become aroused before intercourse the man should meditate on the image of the vulva, or yoni; the woman meditates on the penis, or lingam (see box).*
6 *The man now enters the woman deeply and solidly, using any position. For a while just move slowly, the woman milking and the man thrusting gently.*
8 *Then become still, staring deep into each other's eyes. Imagine yourselves linked at each chakra, particularly the genitals. Imagine your entire genital area surrounded by a pulsing orb of deep red light.*
9 *Synchronize your breathing, slowly and deeply breathing towards your partner's mouth.*
10 *Imagine the energy generated from your genitals spreading up your spines and throughout your entire bodies. Stay like this for as long as is comfortable, if only for a few minutes.*

AROUSAL MEDITATION
★ *Men: picture the yoni as warm, welcoming, moist, soft, and opening and closing like a flower. Concentrate on the soft smell of musk and imagine the sound of a deep heartbeat, a slow rhythm of the earth, the pulse of life.*
★ *Women: visualize the lingam as erect, mentally examining its different textures. The scent to imagine is patchouli. The sound is that of a faster, more insistent throb.*

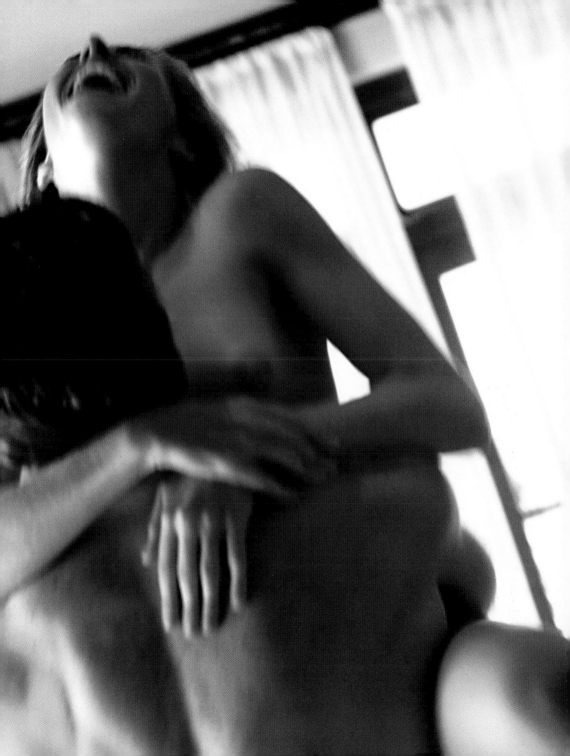

Soothe insomnia

There's nothing worse than not being able to sleep, tossing and turning as you try to switch off for the night. Most insomnia is caused by stress and tension that has accumulated in your mind and body from the day and still remains there when you try to go to sleep. The progressive relaxation technique on these pages irons out the creases and lets you sink into a slumber.

PROGRESSIVE RELAXATION

1 *Sit in bed and think about what is worrying you. Write down a list of your concerns and assure yourself you will deal with them the next day. There is nothing you can do about them at this moment.*

If you find yourself unable to sleep, your mind busy with thoughts, try a couple of drops of White Chestnut remedy from the Bach Flower range.

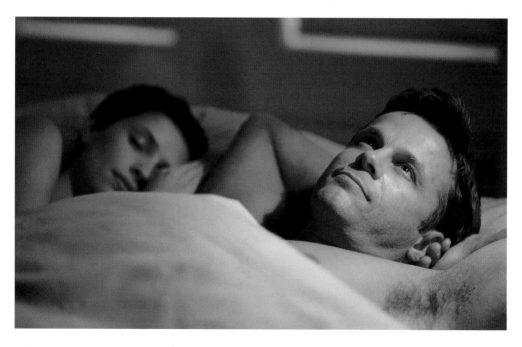

2 *If you are still troubled with thoughts that whirl around in your head, take a couple of drops of Bach White Chestnut remedy.*
3 *Place a few drops of lavender oil on a tissue or handkerchief and tuck it under your head. CAUTION: don't use lavender in early pregnancy.*
4 *Lie down and make yourself comfortable. Become aware of your breathing but don't attempt to change it. Gently close your eyes.*
5 *Become aware of your face and of any tension there. Now contract all the muscles in your face quite forcefully for one or two seconds. Then allow the muscles to relax completely.*
6 *Move now to your neck. Tense and relax. Continue in the same way down through the shoulders and upper arms; the chest and back; the lower arms and hands. Proceed down the body (abdomen, buttocks, thighs, calves, and feet.)*
7 *If you are still feeling tense, repeat the process until you relax.*
8 *Now become aware of your body lying on the bed. Feel it connecting to the earth, being grounded with the earth. Allow any remaining tension to drain off into the earth beneath you.*
9 *If this doesn't work for you, try to imagine lying under the warmth and light of a beautiful, gentle sun (see box, right).*
10 *Give grateful thanks for your body and the wonderful job it does and remind yourself to make time to keep it well nourished, exercised, and relaxed.*
11 *Allow yourself to drift off gently into deep and peaceful sleep.*

IMAGINE THE SUN
Feel the warmth of the sun's rays sink softly into you through every pore in your skin. Sense the soft glow running gently through you like liquid gold. Imagine the sun's healing power cleansing you and filling you with light. Enjoy the feeling of being supported by the earth and caressed by the sun.

Sort out your psyche

Dreams can be a passport to a renewed sense of
creativity, a fresh way of working out tricky problems
and relationships, a means of realizing your deepest
desires and coming to terms with your deepest fears.

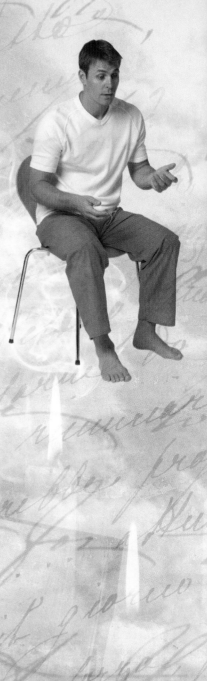

RECALLING YOUR DREAMS

There is no one infallible way to remember dreams.
But there are a few things that seem to help:
■ On waking, it can help to stay lying still in your
sleeping body position to recall your dream.
■ Try saying it aloud or telling someone else your
dream as you wake.
■ Have a "dreambook" or journal by your bed to
write in as soon as you open your eyes. Rewriting
and rereading dreams can add to understanding
them. If you prefer, draw an image that sums up
your dream.
■ Sometimes a simple ritual before sleep, like spending
10 minutes gazing at a candle or into a glass of water,
burning aromatic herbs, or dancing to a favourite piece
of music can help lead you into dreams.

EXPLORING DREAMS, TALKING TO YOUR DREAMS

Try "talking to your dream." Use two chairs or two
cushions. Sit on one and imagine a figure or animal
from your dream is on the other. Try speaking to
the figure or animal, asking it questions. Then switch
seats and speak as if you were the dream replying.
Say whatever comes into your mind, without censoring
it or getting embarrassed. Giving your dream figures
a voice and letting them describe themselves helps
to bring them to the surface. You may be surprised
at what comes up.

Paint or draw your dreams. Look at the techniques for art therapy (see page 118) for ideas on how to free your imagination. If your dream was a frightening nightmare, it might feel safer to put your dream image inside a firm, thick border.

Your image may be a literal picture of what happened in the dream or maybe more of an expression of the mood of the dream through shape and colour. Don't ask other people to "interpret" your painting, although it can be helpful to discuss it with someone else. Ask them what they notice about it.

Use visualization. If a dream ends on an uncertain or disconcerting note, try continuing it in waking time. Relax and do some deep, comfortable breathing and then imagine yourself back in your dream. What might happen next?

Talking to an animal or figure from one of your dreams can have surprising results. Try asking it who it is; what it represents; what message it has for you. Or else, just sit, observe, and listen – it will certainly have important information for you.

Recipes

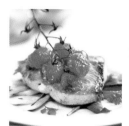
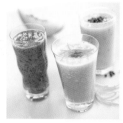
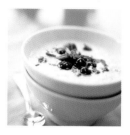
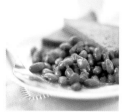

All recipes serve four. Smoothies serve two.

PAN-FRIED FISH

Pan-fry four 6 oz swordfish steaks in 1 tablespoon of hot olive oil. Turn once, and brush the other side with olive oil. They should take about four minutes on each side. At the same time, broil a bunch of cherry tomatoes on the vine, using the highest broiler setting.

Meanwhile put 1 tablespoon of olive oil in another frying pan and heat it. When it's very hot, sear a sliced bunch of scallions (green onions) along with a sliced stick of celery (and any other green vegetables you like). Place each steak on a portion of seared vegetables.

Top with tomatoes, and sprinkle with black pepper and a handful of roughly torn basil leaves.

Why not try salmon or tuna in this way?

SMOOTHIES

Put the ingredients in a blender with a handful of ice cubes, and whip until smooth and creamy.

SUMMER BERRY ATTACK

1 cup each of black-berries, blueberries, and strawberries
1 cup of vanilla-flavored soy milk
ground cinnamon and wild honey to taste (optional)

CARROT SURPRISE

½ cup of carrot juice
½ cup of orange juice
2 cups of pineapple – diced or chopped
2 cups of melon (honeydew or cantaloupe) – chopped

TROPICAL DELIGHT

1 large chopped banana
2 kiwi fruits – peeled and roughly chopped
½ large mango – peeled and chopped
½ large papaya – peeled and chopped
1 cup of freshly squeezed orange juice

OATMEAL

Oatmeal is the simplest breakfast to make. Put ½ cup of oatmeal, and 1½ cups of cold water, per person, in a saucepan.

Bring to a boil and simmer for 4–5 minutes, stirring constantly. Add a handful of black or golden raisins, if you like.

Spoon into a bowl and add your choice of nuts, seeds, chopped banana, or other fruit. If you still need sweetener, add a little maple syrup or honey. Add soy milk to taste.

BAKED BEANS

Place 1 cup of dried navy beans in a pan with 1 quart of water. Bring to a boil and let it boil vigorously for ten minutes. Skim off any foam or scum.

Transfer to an oven-proof dish or bean pot. Add 2 bay leaves, ¼ cup of molasses, and a good sprinkling of black pepper.

Cover tightly and cook slowly in an oven (around 275° F) for about 8 hours (don't let it dry out – check periodically).

Add 5 tablespoons of tomato paste, 6 skinned, chopped tomatoes, and 1 chopped stick of celery. Cook for another two hours. If you leave it overnight it tastes even better!

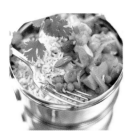 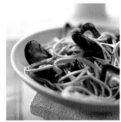 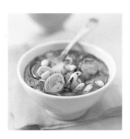 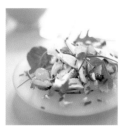

VEGETABLE CURRY

Grind together 1 teaspoon of curry powder, 1 inch of fresh ginger root, 2 garlic cloves, and 1 small onion.

Chop up 3 leeks, 1 small green cabbage, 1½ cups of green beans, 2 carrots, a handful of peas, some cauliflower flowerets and any other vegetables you have at hand.

Fry the ground ingredients in 2 teaspoons of olive oil, and add 1¼ cups of coconut milk (for a low-fat curry, substitute broth for the milk). After it comes to a boil, add the leeks and the other vegetables.

Cook briskly for 10 minutes and add more liquid (hot water – or broth) if needed. Cook according to your preference – whether you like your vegetables crunchy or not.

Serve with rice, and garnish with cilantro (fresh coriander leaves) and roasted almonds.

SEAFOOD STIR-FRY

Chop 1 red pepper, 6 scallions (green onions), 1 garlic clove, 2 cups of button mushrooms, and stir-fry in 1 teaspoon of heated sesame oil.

At the same time, add a large packet of buckwheat noodles to boiling water, turn off the heat, and set aside (they will be ready in about four minutes).

Add soy or fish sauce to stir-fry (according to taste), and 1 tablespoon of water. Add 2 lb of mussels in the shell, plus 1¼ lb of peeled shrimp (and any other seafood you like).

Keep stirring and the mussels will open – discard any that don't. Drain the noodles. When all the mussels have opened, mix the stir-fry with the noodles, and serve.

WHITE BEAN SOUP

In a large pot, heat 2 tablespoons of olive oil. Toss 1 medium, chopped onion in a little olive oil for a few minutes, until soft.

Add 1 large clove of garlic (chopped), 2 drained 14 oz cans of navy beans (small white beans), 2 chopped potatoes, and 2 chopped leeks, and stir before adding 1 quart of chicken or vegetable broth.

Bring to a boil and cook until the potatoes are soft. In a blender or food processor, liquidize half the soup, and return it to the pot. Stir in 1 tablespoon each of fresh parsley and chopped chives. Simmer for three minutes, and serve.

★ Don't worry if you can't find leeks in your local store, Vegetable Curry and White Bean Soup will still taste great without them!

WARM CHICKEN SALAD

Marinate (for an hour at least) four 6 oz skinless chicken breasts in a mixture comprised of 1 tablespoon of toasted sesame oil, 1 tablespoon of freshly squeezed lemon juice, a teaspoon of mustard, and 2 teaspoons of honey, plus a grinding of black pepper. Place in broiler under medium-heat and broil until thoroughly cooked, but still tender.

Meanwhile, make a salad of mixed leaves (include arugula if possible), green grapes (seedless or seed them yourself), pine nuts, chives, celery, and scallions (green onions).

Pile the hot chicken onto the salad ingredients and toss with a dressing made of ¼ cup of lemon juice, 2 tablespoons of white wine vinegar, 1 teaspoon of soy sauce, cracked black pepper, and 1 crushed garlic clove.

Resources

If you want to find out more about the therapies and techniques employed in this book, the following organizations can help. If writing, please send a SASE.

GENERAL
www.alternativemedicine.com
Information on conditions, therapies, and products. Site also lists 17,000 practitioners across the USA.

ALEXANDER TECHNIQUE
NASTAT, PO Box 517
Urbana, IL 61801
nastat@ix.netcom.com
www.alexandertech.com
Tel: (217) 367-6956 or
(800) 473-0620

AROMATHERAPY
American Alliance of
Aromatherapy
PO Box 309
Depoe Bay, OR 97341

National Association for Holistic
Aromatherapy
PO Box 17622
Boulder, CO 80308
info@naha.org
www.naha.org
Tel: (888) ASK-NAHA

AYURVEDA
The National Institute of
Ayurvedic Medicine
584 Milltown Road
Brewster, NY 10509
drgerson@erols.com
www.niam.com
Tel: (914) 278-8700
Fax: (914) 278-8700

BACH FLOWER REMEDIES
Nelson Bach USA, Ltd.
100 Research Drive
Wilmington, MA 01887-4406
Tel: (508) 988-3833 or
(800) 334-0843

BIODANZA
Denise Melo
1104 Willingham Way
Moore, OK 73160
Tel: (405) 794-0500

COLOR THERAPY
The International Association for
Color Therapy
PO Box 3
Potters Bar
Herts EN6 3ET
United Kingdom

DREAM THERAPY
Association for Humanistic
Psychology
45 Franklin Street
Suite 315, San Francisco
CA 94102
www.ahpweb.org
Tel: (415) 864-08850

FENG SHUI
William Spear
24 Village Green Drive
Litchfield, CT 06759
fengshuime@aol.com
Tel: (860) 567-8801

HERBALISM
American Herbalists Guild
PO Box 70
Roosevelt, UT 84066
ahgoffice@earthlink.net
Tel: (435) 722-8434
Fax: (435) 722-8452

HOMEOPATHY
American Institute of
Homeopathy
1585 Glencoe Street
Suite 44, Denver
CO 80220
Tel: (303) 321-4105

MASSAGE
American Massage Therapy
Association
820 Davis Street, Suite 100
Evanston, IL 60201-4444
www.amtamassage.org
Tel: (847) 864-0123
Fax: (847) 864-1178

MEDITATION
American Meditation Institute
PO Box 430, Averill Park
NY 12018
postmaster@americanmeditation.org
www.americanmeditation.org
Tel: (518) 674-8714

NATUROPATHY

American Association of
Naturopathic Physicians
601 Valley Street, Suite 105
Seattle, WA 98109
www.naturopathic.org
Tel: (206) 298-0126
Fax: (206) 298-0129

American Naturopathic Medical
Association
PO Box 96273, Las Vegas
NV 89193
www.webmaster@anma.com
Tel: (702) 897-7053

NUTRITIONAL THERAPY

American Association of
Nutrition Consultants
1641 East Sunset Road
Apt B-117, Las Vegas
NV 89119
Tel: (709) 361-1132

NLP

NLP Seminars Group
International
PO Box 424, Hopatcong
NJ 07843
www.purenlp.com
Tel: (973) 770-3600

POLARITY THERAPY

American Polarity Therapy
Association
PO Box 19858
Boulder, CO 80308
www.polaritytherapy.org
Tel: (303) 545-2080

REBOUNDING

American Institute of
Reboundology
1240 East 800 North
Orem, UT 84097
www.healthbounce.com
Tel: (801) 377-0570

REFLEXOLOGY

International Institute of
Reflexology
PO Box 12642, St Petersburg
FL 33733-2642
www.mitcm.org
Tel: (301) 718-7373 or
       (800) 892-1209
Fax: (301) 718-0735

REIKI

International Center for Reiki
Training
21421 Hilltop Street, Unit #28
Southfield, MI 48034
www.reiki.org
Tel: (800) 332-8112

SHIATSU

American Oriental Bodywork
Therapy Association
50 Maple Street, Manhasset
NY 11030

International School of Shiatsu
10 South Clinton Street
Doylestown, PA 18901
info@shiatsubo.com
www.shiatsubo.com
Tel: (215) 340-9918
Fax: (215) 340-9181

SHYNESS/STRESS

American Counseling
Association
5999 Stevenson Avenue
Alexandria, VI 22304-9800
Tel: (703) 823-0988

SOUND THERAPY

Sound Healers Association
PO Box 2240, Boulder
CO 80306
www.healingsounds.com
Tel: (303) 443-8181
Fax: (303) 443-6023

American Music Therapy
Association, Inc.
8455 Colesville Road
Suite 1000, Silver Spring
MD 20910
info@musictherapy.org
www.musictherapy.org
Tel: (301) 589-3300

TIBETAN HEALING

www.tibetanmedicine.com
Lists practitioners in US and
Canada.

YOGA

International Association of
Yoga Therapists
109 Hillside Avenue,
Mill Valley, CA 94941
Tel: (415) 383-4587

Further reading

GENERAL

Alexander, J., **The Natural Year: A seasonal guide to alternative health and beauty**, Avon Books, 1999
Alexander, J., **Rituals for Sacred Living**, Sterling Pubns, 1999
Murray, M. & Pizzorno, J., **The Encyclopedia of Natural Medicine**, Prima Pubns, 1997
Sullivan, K. (ed.), **The Complete Family Guide to Natural Home Remedies**, Element, 1997

ACUPRESSURE

Harvey, E. & Oatley, M., **Acupressure**, Hodder & Stoughton, 1995
Jarmey, C. & Tindall, J., **Acupressure for Common Ailments**, Fireside, 1991

AFFIRMATION

Hay, L., **You Can Heal Your Life**, Hay House, 1999

ALEXANDER TECHNIQUE

Brennen, R., **Mind & Body Stress Relief with the Alexander Technique**, Thorsons, 1998
MacDonald, G., **The Complete Illustrated Guide to the Alexander Technique**, Element, 1998

AROMATHERAPY

Davies, P., **A-Z of Aromatherapy**, C. W. Daniel, 1999
Worwood, V., **The Fragrant Pharmacy**, Bantam Books, 1991

AYURVEDA

Morningstar, A., **The Ayurvedic Cookbook**, Lotus Light, 1990
Morrison, J., **The Book of Ayurveda**, Fireside, 1995

BACH FLOWER REMEDIES

Ball, S., **Bach Flower Remedies for Men**, C. W. Daniel, 1997
Ball, S., **The Bach Remedies Workbook**, C. W. Daniel, 1998
Howard, J., **Bach Flower Remedies for Women**, C. W. Daniel, 1993

BREATHING

Bennett, B., **Breathing into Life**, HarperSanFrancisco, 1993
Weller, S., **The Breath Book**, Thorsons, 1999

CHI KUNG

Chuen, L., **The Way of Healing**, Broadway Books, 1999
Cohen, K., **The Way of Qigong**, Ballantine Books, 1997

COLOR THERAPY

Chiazzari, S., **The Complete Book of Color**, Element, 1999
Gimbel, T., **Healing with Color and Light**, Fireside, 1994

DETOXING

Alexander, J., **The Detox Plan**, Journey Editions, 1998
MacDonald, S., **Detoxification & Healing**, Keats Publishing, 1997

DREAM THERAPY

Goodison, L., **The Dreams of Women**, Berkley Pub Grp., 1995
Hamilton-Parker, C., **The Hidden Meaning of Dreams**, Sterling Pubns, 1999

FENG SHUI

Alexander, J., **Spirit of the Home**, Thorsons, 1998
Lazenby, G., **The Feng Shui House Book**, Watson-Guptill Pubns, 1998
Shurety, S., **Feng Shui for Your Home**, Trafalgar Square, 1997

HEALTHY HOME

Kruger, A., **H is for ecoHome**, Avon Books, 1992
Logan, K., **Clean House, Clean Planet**, Pocket Books, 1997
Pearson, D., **The Natural House Book**, Fireside, 1996

HOMEOPATHY

Lockie, A. & Geddes, N., **The Family Guide to Homeopathy**, Fireside, 1993

HYDROTHERAPY

Buchman, D., **The Complete Book of Water Therapy**, Keats Publishing, 1994

HYPNOTHERAPY

Peiffer, V., **Thorsons Principles of Hypnotherapy**, Thorsons, 1997
Sheehan, E., **Self-Hypnosis**, Element, 1997

JIN SHIN JYUTSU

Burmeister, A., **Practical Jin Shin Jyutsu**, Thorsons, 1998

MASSAGE

Mitchell, S., **The Complete Illustrated Guide to Massage**, Element, 1999

MEDITATION

Harp, D., **The 3 Minute Meditator**, New Harbinger Pubns, 1996
Kabat-Zinn, J., **Wherever You Go, There You Are**, Hyperion, 1995
Vaughan, S., **Finding the Stillness Within in a Busy World**, C. W. Daniel, 1995

NATUROPATHY

Newman Turner, R., **Naturopathic Medicine**, Thorsons, 1990
Vogel, H., **The Nature Doctor**, Keats Publishing, 1991

NLP

Beaver, D., **NLP for Lazy Learning**, Element, 1998
O'Connor, J. & McDermott, I., **The Principles of NLP**, Thorsons, 1996

NUTRITIONAL THERAPY

Holford, P., **The Optimum Nutrition Bible**, Crossing Press, 1990
Lazarides, L., **The Nutritional Health Bible**, Thorsons, 1998

POLARITY THERAPY

Stone, R., **Health Building**, CRCS Pubns, 1986

REBOUNDING

Wilburn, M., **Starbound**, Orion, 1993 (mail order only: see Resources for address)

REFLEXOLOGY

Ducie, S., **The Self-Help Reflexology Handbook**, Vermilion, 1997
Gillanders, A., **The Joy of Reflexology**, Little, Brown, 1995

REIKI

Honervogt, T., **Reiki**, Owl Books, 1998
Hall, M., **Practical Reiki**, Thorsons, 1997

SHIATSU

Ferguson, P., **The Self-Shiatsu Handbook**, Perigee, 1995
Lundberg, P., **The Book of Shiatsu**, Fireside, 1992

SHYNESS

Crawford, L. & Taylor, L., **Shyness: Your questions answered**, Element, 1998

SOUND THERAPY

Goldman, J., **Healing Sounds**, Element, 1996
Dewhurst-Maddock, O., **The Book of Sound Therapy**, Fireside, 1993

STRESS MANAGEMENT

Peiffer, V., **Principles of Stress Management**, Thorsons, 1997
Wildwood, C., **The Complete Guide to Reducing Stress**, London Bridge Trade, 1997

TANTRA

Anand, M., **The Art of Sexual Magic**, Putnam Pub Group, 1995

TIBETAN HEALING

Donden, Y., **Healing Through Balance**, Snow Lion Pubns, 1986

TIME MANAGEMENT

Price, L., **Coping through Effective Time Management**, Rosen Publishing Group, 1991
Douglass, M. & Douglass, D., **Manage Your Time, Your Work, Yourself**, Amacom, 1993

VISUALIZATION

Graham, H., **Pocket Guide to Visualization**, Crossing Pr, 1997
Wills, P., **Visualization: A beginner's guide**, Hodder & Stoughton, 1999

YOGA

Nagarathna, R., Nagendra, H., & Monro, R., **Yoga for Common Ailments**, Fireside, 1991
Shivapremananda, S., **Yoga for Stress Relief**, Random House, 1998
Weller, S., **Yoga for Long Life**, Thorsons, 1998

Index

A

arguments 78
aromatherapy see essential oils
arousal meditation 146
art therapy 118
Ayurveda, and exercise 120, 121

B

Bach Flower Remedies 77, 78, 84
back strain 43, 64, 65
baths 140–141, 144
bedrooms
    as pleasure zone 132
    as sanctuary 130, 134–135
behaviour, changing 22
Biodanza 116
blues, banishing the 84–85
body language 82–83
breakfasts 27, 30–31, 152
breathing exercises 47, 95
business engagements 80, 92

C

calming 23, 50, 111
    foods 114–115
car 42–43
career boosting 58
centring 23, 111
chakras 100, 101
chi kung 16–17, 48, 75, 98–99
    starting pose 16
clothes, for success 24–25
clutter clearing 42, 56, 130
colds, remedies and baths for
    38–39, 140, 144
colours of workwear 24–25
computer use 65
concentration 68–69
confidence boosters 74–75

cool, keeping your 47, 48–49
cooling breath 95

D

dance therapy 116
desk 55, 58, 60–61
    decluttering 56
    making a shrine 106
detoxing 37, 141
diet 28
    and Tibetan medicine
    122–123
dinner table, intimate 124
disappointment 86–87
dreams 150–151
driving strategies 45, 46
dust mites 134

E

EMFs (electromagnetic fields)
    62, 134, 135
energy
    balancing 50, 126
    boosting 72, 96–97
    foods 92, 114–115
    rebalancing 98–99, 100–101
entrainment 88–89
environment at work 62–63
Epsom salts bath 140
essential oils
    for arguments 78
    for the blues 85
    for hangover 36
    for releasing tension 69
    in work space 57
    massage 136
    soothing/relaxing 48
exercise 18–21, 120–121
eye strain 70–71

F

facial massage 142
feelings, getting in touch with 119
feng shui
    and better bedrooms 130
    and romance 124
    and work 57, 80
food 29, 31
    for moods 114–115
    recipes 152–153
    see also breakfasts, lunch-time
foot massage 138–139

G

GS (geopathic stress) 135
grounding 16

H

hangover zapping 36
healthy eating 28–29
herbalism 34
homeopathy
    for the blues 85
    for colds 39
    for hangover 36
    for sickness/indigestion 34

I

indigestion 34
insomnia 148

J

jet lag 50
jin shin jyutsu 50

L

Liver Flush 37
lunch-time 91, 92–93
lymphatic system 13, 37

M

mantra 23
massage 136, 138–139, 142
meditation exercise 23
memory, foods for 92
mindfulness 45, 51
moods
    changing with music 88–89
    foods for 114–115
    shifting on coming home 110
music therapy 42, 88–89

N

neck strain, at work 64, 65
negotiate with your body 76
NLP (neuro-linguistic
    programming) 22

P

palming meditation 94
passion raiser 145
personal space 83
plants, and pollutants 63
positive affirmations 51
posture 43, 64, 65, 74
power posture 74
power meetings 80
power suit 24
problem resolving 118
progressive relaxation 148–149
psyche 126, 150

R

rapport, in the work place 82–83
rebalancing 96–97, 126–127
rebounding 18–21
recharging your batteries 94
re-energizer, five minute 68–69
refresher postures, basic 72–73

Reiki relaxation 111
relaxation 111, 136, 148–149
revitalization 50, 92
road rage 46
romance 124

S

Salutation to the Sun 14–15
self-confidence 74
senses 83
sensuality, arousing 145
sex 146
shyness 76–77
sick office syndrome 62–63
sitting see posture
skin brushing 13
sleep 140, 148
smoothies 30, 32, 152
sound meditation 100
sound therapy 44
spine see back strain
spiritual emergency kit 42
spiritual symbols 42
steam, for colds 38
stress releases/reduction 47, 50
stretch 12, 14–15, 108–109
subconscious, tapping the 119
success
    dressing for 24–25
    feng shui your desk 57
    programming for 22
supplements, for colds 38
swish technique 22

T

Tantric sex 146
tension releasing 44, 46, 50, 69
    78
thinking ahead 106–107

Three Taps 98–99
Tibetan medicine 122–123
toxins, expelling 13, 37, 141

U

Ujjayi 47

V

verbal language, and rapport 83
visualization techniques
    for arguments 78
    for disappointment 86–87

W

wake-up mind and body 11, 12
winding down 126–127,
    138–139
working day
    attitude to 11
    coping with 98
    end of 105, 106–107
working space 55, 56–57
    see also desk, sick office
    syndrome
writing 119

Y

yoga
    basic refresher postures 72–73
    boost energy levels 96–97
    for relaxing/winding down
        126–127
    hand and foot gymnastics 49
    shoulder-shrugging 49
    stretch away the day 108–109
    Sun Salute 14–15